LOSE IT *for* LIFE

STUDY GUIDE AND
DEVOTIONAL JOURNAL

Stephen Arterburn, M.Ed.

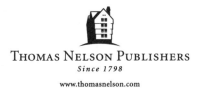

THOMAS NELSON PUBLISHERS
Since 1798

www.thomasnelson.com

Lose It for Life: Study Guide and Devotional Journal

Produced by The Livingstone Corporation (www.LivingstoneCorp.com). Contributing writers: Dana Veerman, Dave Veerman, Linda Washington, and Neil Wilson. Designer: Kirk Luttrell. Compositor: Joel Bartlett.

Printed in the United States of America
06 07 08 RRD 9 8 7 6 5 4 3 2 1

CONTENTS

HOW TO USE THIS BOOK

Congratulations! You are on your way to a new life of freedom and community. You've taken the first step in your healing and weight-loss process by joining this group, and you will not be disappointed.

This book is part of a package to use in your LIFL group. You've received the book *Lose It for Life* and the accompanying audio CDs by Stephen Arterburn, along with this *Study Guide and Devotional Journal*. Over the next eighteen weeks, you will spend time with your group once a week in discussion and prayer.

In each session, you will watch a video from Stephen Arterburn with encouraging stories, scriptural teaching, and helpful insights for your weight-loss journey. After hearing from Steve, you will spend time in your group reading and discussing the material in this study guide. Each week is divided into eight parts:

❖ Introduction

❖ Description of the LIFL Concept for the week

❖ Scripture passage with teaching

❖ Questions to apply the Scripture teaching to life

❖ Case study with questions for individual or group use

❖ A closing thought to challenge you in your journey

❖ Devotional journal space for personal use during the week

❖ Weekly reflection and goals

Each session concludes with a week's worth of daily Bible passages, devotional thoughts, and journaling space. Then you will find a "summary" page where you can chart your journey from the past week and set goals for the week to come.

This should be an exciting time for you. Open up and share with your group. Allow God to use this material to show you areas that need healing and change. With God's help, you really can Lose It for Life.

INTRODUCTION

Black pants held up with suspenders. Striped shirt. Painted white face. Silently, the mime creates a box around himself—an imaginary box, of course. He looks around and finds walls to his right and left, front and back. He's trapped. A look of panic crosses his face. How will he get out?

If you have seen a mime perform, you know that he inevitably finds a way "out." If not, when the performance ends, he simply walks through the imaginary walls.

But let's say this mime continues to stay "trapped" in his imaginary box. His panic is real and he begins to scream (silently, of course). *What is wrong with him?* you wonder. You try to convince him of his illusion, but he continues to push wildly at the imaginary walls. Eventually you give up and leave.

That sounds crazy, but we all do this when we build up walls of misconceptions and rationalizations around us. We may think, for example, "I'm fat because my parents are fat," "There's nothing I can do," or "It's not my fault." We lie to the world and to ourselves so we don't have to take the blame. Like the mime, we build imaginary walls and tell ourselves that we can't escape, we're stuck with the way we are, we're trapped.

VIDEO 1

Notes from video:

_____

_____

_____

_____

_____

_____

_____

_____

_____

_____

_____

LIFL CONCEPT 1

THE PRISONS AND CHAINS THAT TRAP US AND KEEP US FROM A LIFE OF FREEDOM ARE THE ONES WE CREATE FOR OURSELVES.

Rationalizing can become a way of life. We seem to spend most of our lives making excuses. In school, we make up reasons for not finishing our homework. At home, we have excuses about why the plates are still in the sink. At work, we have plenty of circumstances to explain why we are late—again. Excuses are common, and making them will only lead to trouble. We may think we are fooling others, but they usually see right through the deception. We are only fooling ourselves. And when these excuses, these walls, involve weight, this practice can be deadly.

One excuse or one wrong choice does not make someone fat. Obesity usually involves a series of choices. Every meal offers a number of choices—when to eat, what to eat, and how much to eat. Every morning provides the opportunity to choose to exercise or stay in bed. A bad food choice one day won't make a person fat, but consuming bad foods every day and at every meal will.

By continuing to make poor choices and then rationalizing those choices, soon you will be chained to these bad choices and imprisoned by excuses, unable to escape.

How do you become free? The first step is to see that you're in a prison. The second step is to realize who put you there. Here's a clue: It's not your parents, your peers, or compelling marketing by fatty fast food chains. You have put yourself there. You made the wrong choices, and now you are making the excuses.

SCRIPTURE

ROMANS 7:14–25

The law is good, then. The trouble is not with the law but with me, because I am sold into slavery, with sin as my master. I don't understand myself at all, for I really want to do what is right, but I don't do it. Instead, I do the very thing I hate. I know perfectly well that what I am doing is wrong, and my bad conscience shows that I agree that the law is good. But I can't help myself, because it is sin inside me that makes me do these evil things.

I know I am rotten through and through so far as my old sinful nature is concerned. No matter which way I turn, I can't make myself do right. I want to, but I can't. When I want to do good, I don't. And when I try not to do wrong, I do it anyway. But if I am doing what I don't want to do, I am not really the one doing it; the sin within me is doing it.

It seems to be a fact of life that when I want to do what is right, I inevitably do what is wrong. I love God's law with all my heart. But there is another law at work within me that is at war with my mind. This law wins the fight and makes me a slave to the sin that is still within me. Oh, what a miserable person I am! Who will free me from this life that is dominated by sin? Thank God! The answer is in Jesus Christ our Lord. So you see how it is: In my mind I really want to obey God's law, but because of my sinful nature I am a slave to sin.

Real friends tell us things we don't want to hear. That's one of the ways we find out what kind of friend God is—when He tells us things almost no one else will tell us. For example, the Bible passage above begins by reminding us that "the law is good." This means God's moral code isn't arbitrary or optional. God's law is good because it's good for us. And because it is God's law, it is unbreakable. The expression "breaking the law" is misleading. We can ignore a law or be ignorant of a law, but we can't break it. It's closer to the truth to say, "we break ourselves on the law," "we shoot ourselves in the foot," or as LIFL Concept One puts it, "The prisons and chains that trap us and keep us from a life of freedom are the ones we create for ourselves." We may want to spin an excuse or blame others (even God) for the problems in our lives, but Concept One reminds us, like a real friend, that the moment we realize we're stuck is the moment we need to also realize that we've made decisions and taken actions that have led to our "stuck-ness."

The apostle Paul, who penned the words in Romans 7:14–25, revealed his human side in that passage. He wasn't teaching about human problems and challenges that come from the outside. Like us, he was an insider. We may have different personal examples about doing what we don't want to do and not doing what we want to do, but we have no problem understanding what Paul meant. We're in the same predicament as he was.

It's interesting and helpful for us to listen in as this wise person struggles with his failures. He makes the same discoveries we make when we honestly examine our lives, but the conclusion Paul comes to is quite different from the ones many of us reach. The hopeful lesson we can learn from Paul is that, while we must realize we're responsible for where we're stuck; we will remain stuck if we give up, or try to blame others, or even redouble our efforts to get ourselves unstuck by sheer will. Instead, we can follow Paul's example and grab on to the help God offers us in Jesus Christ.

Let's trace Paul's thinking. Earlier in his letter to the Romans, Paul made the case that God's law isn't a "checklist for life" but a standard of life none of us can meet. Because we all start out as sinners and immediately begin sinning as soon as we're able, by the time we find out there is a standard, we've already fallen short of it (Romans 3:23). This jarring realization is like one of those moments when we're driving along and suddenly hear the siren behind us. A glance in the rearview mirror reveals flashing lights. Were we speeding? We can't remember seeing a speed sign. Have we committed some other driving offense? When God's law turns on the siren and lights, we know we're in trouble.

Our run-in with God's law has a lot more consequences than a traffic stop. We can't afford the ticket. We won't get off with a warning. God's law doesn't stop us just to create a problem, but to reveal our problem with sin. The law shows what we've already done. We may resent or fear the interruption, but it's for our good. It confronts us with the truth. Other factors like distractions or the influences of others don't take away the fact that we are at the wheel. The fault comes back to us. And we don't like that. We may get angry or defensive, rationalize, or even indulge in more of the same bad behavior that got the law's attention.

The hardest part to face in all of this is our helplessness. Even the wise step of owning our responsibility confronts us with the question: If we got ourselves into this mess, shouldn't we be able to get ourselves out of it? But we can't. Paul tells us that even though he loved God's law, he realized there was "another law at work within me that is at war with my mind. This law wins the fight and makes me a slave to the sin that is still within me." What a moment of helplessness! Most of us don't reach this point until we've tried hard to work our way, starve our way, and punish our way out of our sin habits. If we don't die trying, we keep coming back to the fork in the road called helplessness. And this can be one of the best moments in life if we take the wise next step: turn away from the way of despair and hopelessness and take the way of help and hope.

Helplessness is not the same thing as hopelessness. Hopelessness is a final destination, ending with despair. It's thinking that we can't help ourselves and that no one else can help us either. With helplessness there's still a lot of room for hope. We can feel helpless to help ourselves yet be filled with hope when we discover someone is able and willing to help us. That's exactly where Paul takes us. "Oh, what a miserable person I am! Who will free me from this life that is dominated by sin? Thank God! The answer is in Jesus Christ our Lord" (Romans 7:24–25).

The first LIFL concept takes us to the starting point: helplessness with hope. We take responsibility not only for our situation but also for getting the help we need from the only one who can ultimately give it—Jesus Christ. In the middle of our helplessness Christ says, "My purpose is to give life in all its fullness" (John 10:10).

DISCUSSION QUESTIONS ABOUT SCRIPTURE

❖ What was Paul's struggle?

_____

_____

_____

_____

_____

_____

❖ If you stopped reading at Romans 7:23, what would you conclude about our human situation?

_____

_____

_____

_____

_____

_____

❖ What hope did Paul offer?

_____

_____

_____

_____

_____

❖ In what ways have you experienced hopelessness in your struggle?

_____

_____

_____

_____

_____

_____

❖ What encouragement do you find in this passage?

_____

_____

_____

_____

_____

_____

_____

_____

❖ What keeps you from losing weight? What walls do you put up?

_____

_____

_____

_____

_____

_____

_____

_____

_____

❖ Based on the insights from this lesson, what steps are you going to take to tear down these walls?

_____

_____

_____

_____

_____

_____

_____

_____

_____

CASE STUDY

BETH

Beth had been told numerous times that she needed to lose weight. She had been gaining steadily and was now obviously obese. When friends encouraged her to go on a diet, she shrugged them off saying that she was just big-boned or that there was "more to love." Beth felt like a failure and knew she would fail again with a new fad diet. So she convinced herself that she didn't have a problem. Plus, she thought, there were other reasons for her condition. Her mother was fat, so she was fat. It was genetics, nothing she could do about it. She couldn't be expected to lose weight.

YOUR TURN

❖ What do Beth's friends think her problem is?

_____

_____

_____

_____

❖ What is Beth's real problem?

_____

_____

_____

_____

❖ What are Beth's prison walls and chains?

_____

_____

_____

_____

❖ What will it take for Beth to break out of her prison?

_____

_____

_____

AS A GROUP

❖ What are some of the prisons and chains people create?

_____

_____

_____

_____

_____

_____

❖ Who, if anyone, has addressed your prisons?

_____

_____

_____

_____

_____

❖ How would you respond to them?

_____

_____

_____

_____

_____

_____

CHALLENGE

We are all trapped in our own prisons. Some are related to weight, some connected to attaining other dreams. We all must take the time to confront our issues, see ourselves as we really are, and, in hope, ask God for help.

Ask Him today to open your eyes and show you your prison. Humble yourself before Him and allow Him to take control of your life. Identify your walls and create a plan of how to tear them down.

What are you going to do today to begin your journey to freedom?

DAILY DEVOTIONAL JOURNAL

DAY 1

Scripture: JEREMIAH 17:7–10

But blessed are those who trust in the LORD and have made the LORD their hope and confidence. They are like trees planted along a riverbank, with roots that reach deep into the water. Such trees are not bothered by the heat or worried by long months of drought. Their leaves stay green, and they never stop producing fruit.

The human heart is the most deceitful of all things, and desperately wicked. Who really knows how bad it is? But I, the LORD, search all hearts and examine secret motives. I give all people their due rewards, according to what their actions deserve.

DEVOTIONAL THOUGHT

What a beautiful word picture this passage gives us: a tree with deep roots, standing strong. God, through His prophet, Jeremiah, is saying that the secret to living well and flourishing is to trust in Him, putting our confidence in Him alone.

Then we hear a contrasting word, a reminder that human nature can deceive us and pull us away from God, if we allow it. So the choice is clear: trust ourselves and we'll wither in the heat. Trust in God, and we'll survive and thrive.

Where are you placing your trust?

TRUTH I WILL FOCUS ON TODAY

_____

_____

_____

_____

MY PRAYER

_____

_____

_____

_____

DAY 2

Scripture: ROMANS 5:3–5

We can rejoice, too, when we run into problems and trials, for we know that they help us develop endurance. And endurance develops strength of character, and character strengthens our confident hope of salvation. And this hope will not lead to disappointment. For we know how dearly God loves us, because he has given us the Holy Spirit to fill our hearts with his love.

DEVOTIONAL THOUGHT

No one has guaranteed that life will be easy. In fact, the opposite is true—life is hard. That's because we live in a sin-broken world where no one is perfect—not even you. Everyone has problems and trials. The issue is not the whether or not we will confront struggles, conflicts, and challenges, but how we will respond when they come. Will we give in or give up? The choice is ours.

Today you will have the same choice, even when you fail. Will you take it as defeat and walk away, or will you see this setback as an opportunity to grow in your faith? It's all about your attitude.

TRUTH I WILL FOCUS ON TODAY

_____

_____

_____

_____

MY PRAYER

_____

_____

_____

_____

DAY 3

Scripture: ROMANS 8:5–10, 12

Those who are dominated by the sinful nature think about sinful things, but those who are controlled by the Holy Spirit think about things that please the Spirit. So letting your sinful nature control your mind leads to death. But letting the Spirit control your mind leads to life and peace. For the sinful nature is always hostile to God. It never did obey God's laws, and it never will. That's why those who are still under the control of their sinful nature can never please God.

But you are not controlled by your sinful nature. You are controlled by the Spirit if you have the Spirit of God living in you. (And remember that those who do not have the Spirit of Christ living in them do not belong to him at all.) And Christ lives within you, so even though your body will die because of sin, the Spirit gives you life because you have been made right with God. . . .

Therefore, dear brothers and sisters, you have no obligation to do what your sinful nature urges you to do.

DEVOTIONAL THOUGHT

Because we are born in sin, we will struggle with sin. But sin does not have to control us. Christ has freed us from our sins, making us free to live to please Him. Sometimes it's a matter of focus. As the text reminds us, "Those who are controlled by the Holy Spirit think about things that please the Spirit."

So where are your thoughts these days? When tempted to make those chains and build those walls, remember this powerful promise: "You have no obligation to do what your sinful nature urges you to do."

TRUTH I WILL FOCUS ON TODAY

_____

_____

_____

_____

MY PRAYER

_____

_____

_____

DAY 4

Scripture: 1 CORINTHIANS 6:12–13A

You say, "I am allowed to do anything"—but not everything is good for you. And even though "I am allowed to do anything," I must not become a slave to anything. You say, "Food was made for the stomach, and the stomach for food."

DEVOTIONAL THOUGHT

Now here's an interesting statement to find in the Bible: "Food was made for the stomach." That may seem obvious, but some people make food much more important than that, becoming obsessed with food and consuming it. That's when food and appetite become the masters, and we become the slaves.

The teaching of this passage is clear. Although we are allowed to do anything (that is, we have the freedom), we should stay away from any specific actions or habits that harm us and do not glorify God. But again, it's our choice. God gives us that freedom.

TRUTH I WILL FOCUS ON TODAY

_____

_____

_____

_____

MY PRAYER

_____

_____

_____

_____

DAY 5

Scripture: GALATIANS 5:16–18

So I say, let the Holy Spirit guide your lives. Then you won't be doing what your sinful nature craves. The sinful nature wants to do evil, which is just the opposite of what the Spirit wants. And the Spirit gives us desires that are the opposite of what the sinful nature desires. These two forces are constantly fighting each other, so you are not free to carry out your good intentions. By when you are directed by the Spirit, you are not under obligation to the law of Moses.

DEVOTIONAL THOUGHT

Are you picking up a theme this week? It's about choices and control. God gives us the freedom to make important choices that can determine the outcome of our lives. He tells us what is right and good for us and urges us to make the right choices, but He leaves the choosing up to us.

Left alone, we would consistently choose wrong. That's because of the pull of our sinful nature. But God, working in us by His Holy Spirit, gives us the power to make good choices, to go the right way. The key is submitting to Him.

TRUTH I WILL FOCUS ON TODAY

_____

_____

_____

_____

MY PRAYER

_____

_____

_____

_____

DAY 6

Scripture: EPHESIANS 4:21–25

Since you have heard about Jesus and have learned the truth that comes from him, throw off your old sinful nature and your former way of life, which is corrupted by lust and deception. Instead, let the Spirit renew your thoughts and attitudes. Put on your new nature, created to be like God—truly righteous and holy.

So stop telling lies. Let us tell our neighbors the truth, for we are all parts of the same body.

DEVOTIONAL THOUGHT

So now we know the truth, about God (He loves us and wants the best for us), about human nature (we are sinners and the downward pull of sin is strong), and about choices (we can choose to "throw off" the old and "put on" the new). That's the truth, and that truth can free us from the chains and prisons built by lies, excuses, and rationalizations. Hold on to the truth!

TRUTH I WILL FOCUS ON TODAY

_____

_____

_____

_____

MY PRAYER

_____

_____

_____

_____

DAY 7

Scripture: JAMES 1:13–16

And remember, when you are being tempted, do not say, "God is tempting me." God is never tempted to do wrong, and he never tempts anyone else. Temptation comes from our own desires, which entice us and drag us away. These desires give birth to sinful actions. And when sin is allowed to grow, it gives birth to death. So don't be misled, my dear brothers and sisters.

DEVOTIONAL THOUGHT

Here's another tough truth—our temptations come from *inside* of us, not outside. The first step in resisting temptation is to recognize that we need help, help from God. Otherwise, we'll follow the natural progression of being enticed and dragged away. So when you feel the pull of temptation, recognize the source and ask God for His power to resist and turn away.

TRUTH I WILL FOCUS ON TODAY

_____

_____

_____

_____

MY PRAYER

_____

_____

_____

_____

WEEKLY PROGRESS AND GOALS

❖ Current weight: _____

❖ Pounds lost this week: _____

NEW INSIGHTS

❖ About myself:

_____

_____

❖ From Scripture:

_____

_____

❖ About weight loss:

_____

_____

PLAN FOR NEXT WEEK

❖ Personal issue to focus on:

_____

_____

❖ Biblical truth to live out:

_____

_____

❖ Food to eliminate or restrict for the week:

_____

_____

❖ Exercise goals:

_____

_____

INTRODUCTION

Walking outside, you quickly put on your sunglasses to block the bright sunlight. The dark lenses dim the strong rays and bring relief to your squinting eyes. Seeing better, you continue on your walk.

Everyone knows how sunglasses work—they shade our vision on a sunny day, darkening our view. But did you know that there are sunglasses for cloudy days? The orange lenses of these sunglasses bring light to our vision and make everything look brighter.

Often we seem to be wearing *orange* sunglasses. Instead of seeing the reality of our weaknesses and sins, we deceive ourselves into thinking that we aren't too bad after all. We put on the orange glasses to brighten our view and keep from confronting our problem areas.

When we fool ourselves this way, we begin to believe a lie. Consider a person's weight, for example. It's easy to overlook the body changes or make excuses instead of facing the situation head on. Life isn't always bright and clear. Sin always darkens our lives, and we only hurt ourselves by pretending that the issues don't exist.

Take off your tinted glasses and see who you really are. Then you will be able to make the necessary changes and move in the right direction.

VIDEO 2

Notes from video:

_____

_____

_____

_____

_____

_____

_____

_____

_____

_____

_____

LIFL CONCEPT 2

OUR BIGGEST CHALLENGE IS SEEING THE REALITY OF OUR LIVES AND TELLING OURSELVES THE TRUTH.

We have often experienced the consequences of lying to others. A child lies to a parent and gets a time out. A teenager lies to a teacher and gets a detention. Lying to a friend leads to hurt and sometimes even a severed relationship. In court, lying while on the witness stand is perjury and punishable under law. But what about when we lie to ourselves? Who serves us the penalty?

We lie to ourselves when we ignore or rationalize a weight problem. We lie to ourselves when we fail to address the hurt afflicted by a loved one and end up feeding the issue. We may not experience the consequences of our lies immediately or see the repercussions, but others do. Lying to ourselves about overeating or eating the wrong foods, for example, will cause us to gain weight—a fact easily observed by all who know us.

Stop lying to yourself. Take off the rationalizing glasses and see the truth. Yes, the truth may hurt. It's not easy to admit that you've allowed your eating to become an issue. It's painful to work through the hurt and failure. But, if you want to find healing, you have to ask God to open your eyes to these lies and begin to address them.

SCRIPTURE

PSALM 19:12–14

How can I know all the sins lurking in my heart?
    Cleanse me from these hidden faults.
Keep your servant from deliberate sins!
    Don't let them control me.
Then I will be free of guilt
    And innocent of great sin.
May the words of my mouth
    and the meditation of my heart
be pleasing to you, O LORD, my rock and my redeemer.

The verses you just read are an unexpected ending to Psalm 19. You will notice the change in focus if you take a moment to read the first eleven verses of the psalm. David, the author, begins his song with a tribute to the way God reveals clues in nature about Himself. The first six verses describe the "glory of God" as it is reflected in the skies, in the order of the universe, and in the sun's daily romp through the heavens.

Everything David sees in nature "speaks" to him about God's craftsmanship, even though no words are used. The quality of the work speaks volumes. Parts of God's creativity remind David of some of the wonderful moments in life, like the joy of a bridegroom or the thrill of a race well run. One of the casualties of a life out of control shows up in our difficulty to sense God's presence in the world around us. If our view of creation has turned drab and lifeless, we can benefit from letting these verses teach our eyes to see what God has done. If we start with the psalm rather than with our most recent disappointing experience, we can begin to notice the grandeur of God in what He has made. Before long, we will be amazed and humbled by the way that God reveals Himself everywhere.

In verse seven, David shifts his eyes from the panoramic view of the universe to a closer view of the page or scroll in his hand. He marvels over God's law—God's Word. Perhaps the thought that "nothing can hide" from the heat of the sun causes David to realize the similar searching qualities of God's Word. In Psalm 19:7–11, David points out five benefits and three qualities of God's Word. Just as the creation can give us glimpses of God's glory, so His law offers us healthy input that revives our souls, makes us wiser, brings us joy, gives us insight into life, and warns us of dangers. Taking God's Word to heart produces "great rewards." God's Word can do this because of its qualities of fairness, desirability, and sweetness. Exposure to God's Word that leads to correction or encouragement reminds us that God has provided it to us for our good. Whether it tastes like medicine or dessert, it's good for us.

Here, David suddenly turns personal. We can guess at his experience in writing the psalm. As he thinks deeply about the powerful witness that the creation mimes about God and that God gives through His Word, David is surprised by his own inadequacy. The more he gets a clear view of God's greatness, the clearer the view of his own tendencies toward sin becomes. This reality instantly generates another change in the psalm. David stops talking to his human audience and begins speaking to God. Praise gives way to prayer. Comments about "the Lord" turn into humble requests directed *to* the Lord—warn me, cleanse me, and keep me!

The LIFL second concept states: "Our biggest challenge is seeing the reality of our lives and telling ourselves the truth." David's approach in this psalm highlights two truths. *First, learning to see and speak the truth to ourselves begins with learning the truth about God.* The less we know about God, the less we know about ourselves. By choosing to focus his mind on God and God's Word, David was setting himself up for a renewed and truthful look at himself. By looking first at God, David was deliberately putting on truth-tinted glasses he could then use to see his own life. David's approach is worth imitating!

Second, we hide behind three curtains by not telling ourselves the truth: unconscious ("lurking") sins, "hidden" sins, and deliberate sins. The lurking sins are sins of attitude and action that are so ingrained or deep-seated that we don't even recognize them as sin unless someone points them out to us. But the idea of allowing someone else to reveal the sins they see in us can be terrifying. Though we may not know all these sins, we can trust God, who knows them all.

The "hidden" sins are shame and behavior issues that we know are sinful but refuse to acknowledge because the truth will hurt. Unlike the unconscious sins, we know about these hidden sins but aren't sure what to do with them. In David's words, we need them "cleansed." The deliberate sins are the ones we know we're going to do but know we shouldn't do and then do them anyway. Sometimes these sins include the presumptuous conclusion that since God is a forgiving God, it might even be our duty to sin at will so that God will be able to do something He enjoys doing. But the glaring problem with this attitude—premeditated repentance (I'll do this and then tell God I'm sorry)—is that it is not genuine repentance. That attitude deeply disrespects God and endangers our soul. In fact, we can't begin to repent about the sinful behavior until we repent for taking forgiveness for granted.

David arrived at the truth about himself by "walking" through truth about God and His Word. We can follow that same path. And once we begin to see the truth about the sad and ugly sins in ourselves, we can continue to use David's strategy. Note the humility in the final, surprising thoughts of this psalm. It's a prayer that looks forward, saying, in effect, God, where do we go from here? David trusts God to prevent sins from controlling him. He knows it will leave him "free from guilt and innocent of great sin." This psalm is a perfect example of the prayer in the last verse: "May the words of my mouth and the meditation of my heart be pleasing to you, O Lord, my rock and my redeemer."

Accept the challenge of seeing and telling yourself the truth by starting with God and seeking His help every day.

DISCUSSION QUESTIONS ABOUT SCRIPTURE

❖ What are the differences between "lurking sins" and "hidden sins"?

_____

_____

_____

_____

_____

_____

❖ How do those two types of sin differ from "deliberate sins"?

_____

_____

_____

_____

_____

_____

❖ What are some "hidden" sins?

_____

_____

_____

_____

_____

_____

❖ How do we hide our sins?

_____

_____

_____

_____

_____

_____

❖ Why do we lie to ourselves?

_____

_____

_____

_____

_____

❖ Who do you trust to point out your "lurking" sins and tell you the truth?

_____

_____

_____

_____

_____

❖ How would knowing the truth about your sins help you change?

_____

_____

_____

_____

_____

CASE STUDY

TOM

"You're gaining more weight. You really need to watch what you eat." Tom seemed to be hearing those words almost daily from family and friends. But he didn't see the problem. Tom reasoned that he had been overweight his entire life and had managed to survive so far. So what was the issue?

Recently, Tom visited his doctor because his knees had been hurting. There, Tom learned that these new pains could be traced directly to his increased weight. Tom dismissed the doctor's diagnosis and wrote it off to old age. What did his weight have to do with knee problems?

Tom is sick of hearing how he needs to change, so he keeps away from friends. He spends his time at home or doing things alone. He thinks that at forty-two years of age he should know what foods to eat. *Besides, one more donut won't hurt me*, he thinks.

YOUR TURN

❖ Why does Tom struggle with his weight gain?

_____

_____

_____

_____

_____

_____

❖ What is his "lurking" sin?

_____

_____

_____

_____

_____

❖ What could his friends and family do to help?

_____

_____

_____

_____

_____

❖ How has Tom worn the rationalization glasses?

_____

_____

_____

_____

_____

AS A GROUP

❖ In what areas do you tend to be dishonest with yourself?

_____

_____

_____

_____

❖ When do you most likely ignore your own sin?

_____

_____

_____

_____

❖ What are your favorite rationalizations/excuses?

_____

_____

_____

_____

❖ In what other areas—in addition to weight loss—do people rationalize?

_____

_____

_____

_____

CHALLENGE

If you look in a mirror, you should be able to get a fairly accurate look at your face. You'll know if your face is clean and your hair combed. But you won't see your face clearly if the lights are off, if the mirror is wavy or cracked, or if you're wearing the wrong glasses. And doing that would be foolish indeed. Yet that's how we often look at our own shortcomings and sins. Instead of fooling ourselves, we need to look through "truth-tinted" glasses. This means being open to the insight and input of those who know us best. This week, take an honest look at yourself. Ask those whom you trust to offer their insights and suggestions.

DAILY DEVOTIONAL JOURNAL

DAY 1

Scripture: PSALM 119:29

Keep me from lying to myself; give me the privilege of knowing your instructions.

DEVOTIONAL THOUGHT

God knows us thoroughly. He loves us and wants the very best for us. No wonder this psalm writer calls knowing God's instructions a "privilege." His instructions are perfect and perfectly suited for us. He would never lead us astray. And what a profound prayer—"Keep me from lying to myself." Make that your prayer, and ask God to give you His instructions.

TRUTH I WILL FOCUS ON TODAY

_____

_____

_____

_____

MY PRAYER

_____

_____

_____

_____

DAY 2

Scripture: MATTHEW 7:1–5

Do not judge others, and you will not be judged. For you will be treated as you treat others. The standard you use in judging is the standard by which you will be judged.

And why worry about a speck in your friend's eye when you have a log in your own? How can you think of saying to your friend, "Let me help you get rid of that speck in your eye," when you can't see past the log in your own eye? Hypocrite! First get rid of the log in your own eye; then you will see well enough to deal with the speck in your friend's eye.

DEVOTIONAL THOUGHT

One of the reasons we judge others is to take the focus off ourselves. If we can highlight someone else's failures and mistakes, then, perhaps, no one will notice ours. Yet our problems and sins (the "logs") impair our vision and make it virtually impossible to actually help anyone else. How much better to first remove the log!

Ask God to show you the logs in your life—with an honest assessment of yourself—and to help you get them out and move on.

TRUTH I WILL FOCUS ON TODAY

_____

_____

_____

_____

MY PRAYER

_____

_____

_____

_____

DAY 3

Scripture: 1 JOHN 1:8

If we say we have no sin, we are only fooling ourselves and refusing to accept the truth.

DEVOTIONAL THOUGHT

How many times do you sin every day? Every hour? Every minute? Let's face it—sin is part of our lives. We were born sinners, and our natural desires are turned in that direction. Why is it, then, that we find it easy to gloss over our sins, to ignore them, or to rationalize them away? When we do that, we are only "fooling ourselves."

The first step to seeing the truth is to stop believing the lie. Look at yourself honestly, as a sinner who desperately needs God's help.

TRUTH I WILL FOCUS ON TODAY

_____

_____

_____

_____

MY PRAYER

_____

_____

_____

_____

DAY 4

Scripture: JOHN 8:32

You will know the truth, and the truth will set you free.

DEVOTIONAL THOUGHT

This is one of the most quoted verses in the Bible. It appears, in fact, in the lobby of the CIA building. Usually, it is used to illustrate the importance of discovering the truth and highlighting the fact that knowing truth leads to freedom. That fact is *true*, but it's not the point of the verse.

When Jesus made this statement, He was speaking about Himself. Just a couple of sentences later He said, "If the Son [Jesus] sets you free, you will indeed be free" (John 8:36).

Jesus is the truth (see John 14:6), and He can help us see the truth about ourselves, life, and eternal life. So if you want freedom, look to Christ—the Truth.

TRUTH I WILL FOCUS ON TODAY

MY PRAYER

DAY 5

Scripture: JOHN 16:13

When the Spirit of truth comes, he will guide you into all truth.

DEVOTIONAL THOUGHT

In this passage, Jesus told His followers about the Holy Spirit, the "Spirit of truth," who would come. Jesus had been living *with* them, but the Holy Spirit would live *in* them. This means that anyone who has placed his or her trust in Christ as Savior has received the Holy Spirit and has His power available—power to know the truth and to change, from the inside out.

Think about it—God is living in you. He wants to transform you into the kind of person who will glorify Him in all you say and do. You have His power at your disposal.

TRUTH I WILL FOCUS ON TODAY

_____

_____

_____

_____

MY PRAYER

_____

_____

_____

_____

DAY 6

Scripture: PROVERBS 27:6

Wounds from a sincere friend are better than many kisses from an enemy.

DEVOTIONAL THOUGHT

The truth can hurt, especially when someone points out a character flaw or confronts us about a wrong action. But when someone who cares about us and wants only to help us speaks those truths, we should listen carefully and not resent the message or the messenger. We may feel wounded, but those truthful wounds will help us heal.

What friend will speak the truth to you? Will you be open to that friend's words?

TRUTH I WILL FOCUS ON TODAY

_____

_____

_____

_____

MY PRAYER

_____

_____

_____

_____

DAY 7

Scripture: PROVERBS 8:6–7

Listen to me! For I have excellent things to tell you. Everything I say is right, for I speak the truth and detest every kind of deception.

DEVOTIONAL THOUGHT

In this passage, "wisdom" is the one speaking, "Listen to me!" The point is clear: the wise person speaks the truth and hates deception, *every kind*. This includes self-deception, the lies we tell ourselves when we rationalize our behavior and minimize our sins.

A wise person faces the truth squarely and lives accordingly. How wise are you?

TRUTH I WILL FOCUS ON TODAY

_____

_____

_____

_____

MY PRAYER

_____

_____

_____

_____

WEEKLY PROGRESS AND GOALS

❖ Current weight: _____

❖ Pounds lost this week: _____

NEW INSIGHTS

❖ About myself:

_____

_____

❖ From Scripture:

_____

_____

❖ About weight loss:

_____

_____

_____

PLAN FOR NEXT WEEK

❖ Personal issue to focus on:

_____

_____

❖ Biblical truth to live out:

_____

_____

❖ Food to eliminate or restrict for the week:

_____

_____

❖ Exercise goals:

_____

_____

_____

INTRODUCTION

I can do it by myself!" Most parents of three-year-olds have heard that statement. Children know that Mom or Dad would help in a second, but they want to have control. Watching the struggle, the parent leans in to help, only to be pushed away through angry tears. "I can do it on my own!"

Adults can act that way too, insisting on control and doing it their way. Of course, we *should* do some things by ourselves. But often we need help, big time. And that's when refusing outside assistance is foolish, especially from our heavenly Father. In those struggles, we may convince ourselves that we can do it on our own—begin an exercise program, eat better, and establish other healthy habits. As we struggle, deep down inside we know that God can help us, but like small children, we push Him away.

Society tells us to be strong, independent, and never ask for help. We would rather live in our own false ways than allow God to work. Clinging tightly to our lifestyles, we never let go and allow God to change and heal us. But only when we release our stubborn pride and ask God for help will the healing process begin.

VIDEO 3

Notes from video:

_____

_____

_____

_____

_____

_____

_____

_____

_____

_____

_____

LIFL CONCEPT 3

WE WILL NEVER ALLOW FOR CHANGE OR INVITE HEALING INTO OUR LIVES UNTIL WE RECOGNIZE AND RELEASE OUR STUBBORN RESISTANCE.

Imagine that while driving with a friend you become lost on a country road. Nothing looks familiar—no road signs or landmarks to give you a hint of where you are and where to go. "Corn on the right and beans on the left! Keep going this way," you announce confidently to your friend. Refusing to admit that you are lost, you don't even consider stopping for directions. So you just keep driving quickly to who knows where, getting more and more disoriented.

Hearing a story like that we may think, *How foolish!* People should ask for directions, right? But they don't. Yet similar scenes are played out every day in many areas of our lives.

What keeps *us* from asking for help? One barrier is pride. We want to project the image that we are competent and in control. Asking for help would be a sign of weakness, we think, and we don't want anyone to think we can't handle what life gives us. We refuse to admit that something might be wrong. Another barrier is fear—fear that others will think less of us and maybe reject us. Or we may simply be afraid that others will discover the truth about us, that we're not all we have been pretending to be.

These barriers, especially our fear of possible rejection from friends and loved ones, can keep us from growing deeper relationships and from forming new ones. Instead of allowing people in, we hold them at arm's length. But pushing friends away brings no comfort, only loneliness. We know we need to change, but it seems impossible. The risk seems too great.

If that's how you are feeling right now, let go and let God begin to heal you. Ask Him to show you your resistant areas and then give them over to Him. It may be scary, but it's well worth the risk.

SCRIPTURE

ACTS 10:9–16

The next day as Cornelius's messengers were nearing the town, Peter went up on the flat roof to pray. It was about noon, and he was hungry. But while a meal was being prepared, he fell into a trance. He saw the sky open, and something like a large sheet was let down by its four corners. In the sheet were all sorts of animal, reptiles, and birds. Then a voice said to him, "Get up, Peter; kill and eat them."

"No, Lord," Peter declared. "I have never eaten anything that our Jewish laws have declared impure and unclean."

But the voice spoke again: "Do not call something unclean if God has made it clean." The same vision was repeated three times. Then the sheet was suddenly pulled up to heaven.

God gives us many good gifts, including food. The apostle James talked about God's gifts: "Whatever is good and perfect comes down to us from God our Father, who created all the lights in the heavens. He never changes or casts a shifting shadow" (James 1:17). In Peter's unusual vision, God offered some new gifts and Peter didn't know what to do with them.

In our discussion of Concept One we discovered that most of our deepest struggles are self-made. Concept Two showed us that our problems get reinforced because we can't "see" them truthfully. Until we apply these two concepts, we have a distorted view of life. We elevate the trivial and devalue what's really important. For example, we can accept God's good gifts but put them to negative use. God's gift of food can remind us of God's generosity, but food should never take on godlike importance for us. The Giver should be our focus. His gifts are optional benefits. All other hungers should take a back seat to our spiritual hunger for the One who made us. But we allow other desires to drive our actions rather than our deepest need for God. No wonder our lives travel erratically! We were designed to take directions only from the One we know has our ultimate good in mind. At this point we need to experience the truth of Concept Three: "We will never allow for change or invite healing into our lives until we recognize and release our stubborn resistance."

"Stubborn resistance" can refer to a mixture of at least two reactions we have when we discover our actions are creating problems for us. First, we may just grit our teeth over the principle of the thing—no one is going to tell us we're wrong or what to do. We reject guidance and help from just about every source. We might even resist by partial agreement, thinking, "Fine! If you say I got myself into this problem, then I'll get myself out of it!"

Second, we can deny our stubborn resistance by coming up with explanations and excuses for the way we are behaving. We may even try to blame God for the choices we're making.

In Peter's situation up on the rooftop waiting for dinner, the issue quickly became, "Will I obey what God is telling me? In other words, would Peter stick with what was traditional and familiar or carry out this new thing God had said?

In Peter's day, religious Jews defined themselves by dietary rules. Talk about strict! They made a religion out of the saying, "You are what you eat." The guidelines God laid out for His people in the wilderness back in the days of Exodus had become fine-tuned dietary laws that controlled people's daily lives. Peter couldn't imagine eating something that wasn't kosher, even when God invited him to do so in the vision.

The conflict wasn't over what Peter would or wouldn't eat. The real issue was that Jews in Peter's day tended to use the dietary rules as a measuring tape of spirituality. If certain foods were "unclean" and to be avoided, then certain *people* were also "unclean" and to be avoided. Those who had been brought up in Peter's culture thought of Gentiles as unclean and unworthy of God's attention. God used the vision of "unclean" animals to alert Peter to the fact that thoughtless obedience to rules sometimes leads us to ignoring even more important rules.

Peter was invited to go to the house of Cornelius, a Roman Gentile. The standards of the day called for Peter to ignore the invitation and not return an RSVP. That was the safe, expected, and sure-to-be-approved response. But it was not the response that God wanted from Peter. The temptation for Peter would be to stay "stubbornly resistant" to anything other than what he was used to doing. But God was preparing Peter for radical and uncomfortable cooperation with God's plans that even seemed to break some of God's past rules. We know this was a training process because even after this incident, Peter continued to struggle in his relationships with other Jews and their standards on the one hand and with Gentiles on the other. In the letter to the Galatians (2:11–16), Paul reports that he had to confront Peter over Peter's apparent tendency to treat Gentiles as second-class citizens among followers of Christ.

How do we move from a rooftop vision in Joppa to the truth of Concept Three? All of us live by following conscious and unconscious rules and patterns. Even people whose lives are in chaos are behaving under patterns they may not even recognize. These concepts may even appear good or harmless, but they can have a negative flip side.

"Never hurt another person" can become a nightmare if we apply it to mean, "Never say no or disagree with another person because it might hurt his feelings." A good general rule can become tyrannical if not applied thoughtfully. Unfortunately, we tend to be stubbornly resistant to examining the rules we live by. Our repeated patterns may be getting us in trouble, but we find it hard to give them up. They are familiar even if deadly. But until we consider that our rules may be wrong, or that we may be applying them in the wrong way, we are not going to ask for the help we desperately need.

Acts 10 tells us how Peter broke rules and did something great for God and a lot of other people. It wasn't easy to set aside old habits and ingrained attitudes. But almost as soon as he did, good things began to happen! One of the biggest steps you'll take in applying the LIFL concepts will be deciding not to resist stubbornly when you see the truth.

DISCUSSION QUESTIONS ABOUT SCRIPTURE

❖ What was the purpose of the sheet lowered from heaven, filled with animals?

_____

_____

_____

_____

_____

_____

❖ What was Peter's immediate response?

_____

_____

_____

_____

_____

_____

❖ What is "stubborn resistance"?

_____

_____

_____

_____

_____

_____

❖ Why is it so difficult to "let go"?

_____

_____

_____

_____

_____

_____

❖ What keeps you from asking for guidance and help?

_____

_____

_____

_____

_____

_____

_____

_____

❖ What fears do you suspect may be keeping you trapped in unhealthy habits?

_____

_____

_____

_____

_____

_____

_____

_____

❖ As a response to this passage, what ingrained attitudes and patterns are you going release to God?

_____

_____

_____

_____

_____

_____

_____

_____

CASE STUDY

MARY

The weight snuck up on Mary. She wasn't trying to eat her way out of a problem, she just couldn't say no to friends. Mary's issue was a social one. Never wanting to rock the boat, she would simply agree to eat whatever someone offered to her. She was just trying to be considerate.

The calories from the creamy soups, thick burgers, crispy fries, and decadent chocolate desserts eventually caught up with Mary. The late night movies with super-buttered popcorn didn't help. But what could she do? She was afraid that not eating with her friends would be interpreted as judging them. So she joined them in their revelry.

Mary's people-pleasing demeanor kept her from doing what was right for herself physically. She allowed others to influence her decisions instead of considering her own needs. The fear of offending her friends kept Mary from making a healthy decision. What if they didn't want to be her friends anymore?

YOUR TURN

❖ What caused Mary to gain weight?

_____

_____

_____

_____

❖ What are Mary's worries?

_____

_____

_____

_____

❖ What steps does Mary need to take to stop the harmful cycle?

_____

_____

_____

_____

AS A GROUP

❖ How do we allow our fears to control us?

_____

_____

_____

_____

_____

_____

❖ What drives your fears? Why is acknowledging and rejecting our fears worth the risk?

_____

_____

_____

_____

_____

_____

❖ Where do you need to "let go"?

_____

_____

_____

_____

_____

CHALLENGE

It's amazing how stubborn we can be sometimes, especially in revealing weaknesses or asking for help. Consequently, like a child struggling with a simple task or a driver wandering the countryside, we reject answers and push away guidance. Whether motivated by pride or fear, our stubborn resistance prevents us from changing and being healed.

What is keeping you from opening up and reaching out? Let go of those resistant attitudes and take an important step toward healing.

DAILY DEVOTIONAL JOURNAL

DAY 1

Scripture: EXODUS 9:7

Pharaoh sent his officials to investigate, and they discovered that the Israelites had not lost a single animal! But even so, Pharaoh's heart remained stubborn, and he still refused to let the people go.

DEVOTIONAL THOUGHT

You remember the story. God sent Moses to deliver His people from slavery in Egypt. Moses continually went before Pharaoh to ask for the Israelites' freedom. Pharaoh continually, stubbornly refused—some translations say that he "hardened his heart." Eventually, he became so hardened in his stubbornness, that God, in effect, said, "Have it your way," and hardened Pharaoh's heart even more (Exodus 9:12). Stubborn pride can become so ingrained in a person's actions, that he or she can become blinded to terrible realities (as Pharoah was blinded to the plagues).

When do you tend to harden your heart? Ask God to break through your stubbornness and do His softening work.

TRUTH I WILL FOCUS ON TODAY

_____

_____

_____

_____

MY PRAYER

_____

_____

_____

_____

DAY 2

Scripture: **DEUTERONOMY 9:6**

You must recognize that the LORD your God is not giving you this good land because you are good, for you are not—you are a stubborn people.

DEVOTIONAL THOUGHT

In this case, it is not Pharaoh or the Egyptians who are described as "stubborn," but God's chosen people. Instead of trusting in God who had promised them the land, they believed the negative report of ten spies and refused to step forward in faith. Moses confronted them with their true character—not goodness but stubbornness, and this stubbornness would keep them from enjoying the Promised Land.

What a great lesson for us today. God has given us marching orders and has promised His presence and power as we go. Yet too often we listen to the rumors and lies of others and stop in our tracks. What has God told you to do? What's stopping you from doing it?

TRUTH I WILL FOCUS ON TODAY

_____

_____

_____

_____

MY PRAYER

_____

_____

_____

_____

DAY 3

Scripture: PSALM 81:12

So I let them follow their own stubborn desires, living according to their own ideas.

DEVOTIONAL THOUGHT

This passage reflects on the Israelites' wilderness experience. God is saying that because His people insisted on going their own direction and living their own way, He permitted them to do so—leading to their eventual downfall.

We shouldn't think that God approves of how we live simply because things seem to be going well at the moment or that we are feeling okay. God knows us perfectly and only He can see the future. It makes sense to trust Him and follow His lead, regardless of how things look or feel right now.

Don't be blind and stubborn. Open your eyes and follow the Lord.

TRUTH I WILL FOCUS ON TODAY

_____

_____

_____

_____

MY PRAYER

_____

_____

_____

_____

DAY 4

Scripture: ACTS 7:51

You stubborn people! You are heathen at heart and deaf to the truth. Must you forever resist the Holy Spirit? That's what your ancestors did, and so do you!

DEVOTIONAL THOUGHT

In his powerful speech to the Sanhedrin, Stephen blasted his listeners for their stubborn pride that was keeping them from hearing the truth. Even worse, he continued, they were resisting God.

When have you allowed pride to close you off from the truth about yourself? What steps can you take to be open to truth, from God and from others?

TRUTH I WILL FOCUS ON TODAY

_____

_____

_____

_____

MY PRAYER

_____

_____

_____

_____

DAY 5

Scripture: PROVERBS 16:18

Pride goes before destruction, and haughtiness before a fall.

DEVOTIONAL THOUGHT

This familiar proverb highlights a fact that we see played out daily: the cocky, trash-talking athlete who chokes in the big game, the overly confident salesperson who takes a client for granted and loses a customer, the complacent student who fails the final exam. Our falls can be hard and painful. Knowing the truth of this verse intellectually and through painful experience, still we battle the enemy of pride continually. And in some areas of life, losing the battle can be deadly. Ask God to reveal your pride points, and ask Him for humility.

TRUTH I WILL FOCUS ON TODAY

_____

_____

_____

_____

MY PRAYER

_____

_____

_____

_____

DAY 6

Scripture: PROVERBS 28:14

Blessed are those who fear to do wrong, but the stubborn are headed for serious trouble.

DEVOTIONAL THOUGHT

This passage says that a having a healthy fear of doing wrong is the opposite of stubbornness. The idea is that those who are sensitive to the Holy Spirit's voice know when they are headed in the wrong direction or are doing something that is wrong. Then, in obedience, they turn away and move forward on the right path.

Stubborn pride can cause us to refuse to ask for help, even from God. But that leads to "serious trouble." Ask God to give you a tender conscience, with a heart and mind in tune with His desires.

TRUTH I WILL FOCUS ON TODAY

_____

_____

_____

_____

MY PRAYER

_____

_____

_____

_____

DAY 7

Scripture: 2 TIMOTHY 1:7

For God has not given us a spirit of fear and timidity, but of power, love, and self-discipline.

DEVOTIONAL THOUGHT

Here Paul is writing to young Timothy, his protégé, encouraging him to be strong in his convictions and ministry. Paul knew that Timothy could be timid and that he might let his fears keep him from doing what he should.

Fear can paralyze us—fear for safety, or fear of what others might think. Fearing other peoples' opinions often stems from pride. We want to keep up a certain image and are afraid they might learn what we're really like.

Don't allow fear, especially fear of what others think, to keep you from doing what is right and what you should do.

TRUTH I WILL FOCUS ON TODAY

_____

_____

_____

_____

MY PRAYER

_____

_____

_____

_____

WEEKLY PROGRESS AND GOALS

❖ Current weight: _____

❖ Pounds lost this week: _____

NEW INSIGHTS

❖ About myself:

_____

_____

❖ From Scripture:

_____

_____

❖ About weight loss:

_____

_____

PLAN FOR NEXT WEEK

❖ Personal issue to focus on:

_____

_____

❖ Biblical truth to live out:

_____

_____

❖ Food to eliminate or restrict for the week:

_____

_____

❖ Exercise goals:

_____

_____

INTRODUCTION

Sore muscles, purple toenails, chapped legs and arms—these are all evidence that a person is training for a marathon. After four months and hundreds of miles of preparing, the runner crosses the finish line with other runners, out of breath and totally spent, but flashing a huge smile. The pain of her workouts and the race itself was a price gladly paid for the feelings of accomplishment and joy of reaching her goal.

How did this woman get from sitting on the couch to running 26.2 miles? Did she just wake up that morning and decide to go run the marathon? No, she invested hours and hours of training. Sleeping late was no longer an option. She suffered through early morning runs before work and the soreness that followed. Was it worth it? Ask any marathoner that question and you'll hear a resounding "Yes!" The change in habits to reach the goal—the finish line—was worth all the pain.

What difference do you want to see in your life? What price are you willing to pay to reach your goal? What are you willing to suffer to make the desired changes? Just as with athletic training, gain often comes with pain. But the results are well worth the hard work and sacrifice.

VIDEO 4

Notes from video:

_____

_____

_____

_____

_____

_____

_____

_____

_____

_____

LIFL CONCEPT 4

IN ORDER TO CHANGE, WE HAVE TO REPLACE OUR DESIRE TO COMFORT OURSELVES AT ALL COSTS WITH A WILLINGNESS TO SUFFER JUST AS CHRIST SUFFERED FOR US.

"Suffer? I don't want to suffer—count me out." There's a great aversion to suffering in the twenty-first century. We expect things to be easy and are frustrated when anything penetrates our comfort zone. But, there is no easy way to lose weight—to make the pounds suddenly go away. That's a fact of life.

Reaching a worthy goal always requires sacrifice. The business executive sacrifices sleep and endures continual travel to reach the top of the corporate ladder. A pregnant woman experiences great discomfort and pain in pregnancy and birth in order to have a child. A doctor or dentist inflicts pain to bring about healing. The basketball player runs ladder sprints at every practice for a peak performance in the game. The artist spends countless hours of eye and muscle strain crafting a masterpiece.

The greatest example of sacrifice is Jesus. He paid the ultimate price, giving His life for us to provide forgiveness, salvation, and heaven.

Comfort is fine, but making important life changes will mean moving out of our comfort zones. Losing weight requires sacrifice and some pain. This is counterintuitive, but it's true that discomfort and pain often lead to healing and peace. You won't suffer forever. The goal is attainable. Just be prepared to do what you must, enduring the pain, and you'll gain the prize.

SCRIPTURE

JOHN 12:20–32

Some Greeks who had come to Jerusalem for the Passover celebration paid a visit to Philip, who was from Bethsaida in Galilee. They said, "Sir, we want to meet Jesus." Philip told Andrew about it, and they went together to ask Jesus.

Jesus replied, "Now the time has come for the Son of Man to enter into his glory. I tell you the truth, unless a kernel of wheat is planted in the soil and dies, it remains alone. But its death will produce many new kernels—a plentiful harvest of new lives. Those who love their life in this world will lose it. Those who care nothing for their life in this world will keep it for eternity. Anyone who wants to be my disciple must follow me, because my servants must be where I am. And the Father will honor anyone who serves me.

"Now my soul is deeply troubled. Should I pray, 'Father, save me from this hour'? But this is the very reason I came! Father, bring glory to your name."

Then a voice spoke from heaven, saying, "I have already brought glory to my name, and I will do so again." When the crowd heard the voice, some thought it was thunder, while others declared an angel had spoken to him.

Then Jesus told them, "The voice was for your benefit, not mine. The time for judging this world has come, when Satan, the ruler of this world, will be cast out. And when I am lifted up from the earth, I will draw everyone to myself."

A man stopped at a stop sign and the car behind him plowed into his rear bumper, demolishing most of the rear end of the vehicle. Surprised and angry, the man leaped from his car and marched back to the car that had just smashed his. He couldn't believe his eyes. The other driver was sitting calmly in his car, smiling. The man angrily demanded an explanation, "Why did you bang into my car? Can't you see all the damage you've done?"

"Well, yes," the other man responded. "But if you notice, your bumper sticker clearly states, 'If it feels good, do it.' I thought smashing your car would feel good, so I did it. And it did."

We've all run into statements that at first make sense until we actually try to live them out. People who grew up in the 1960s had their own favorite bumper stickers. "Question Authority" was a big seller. But taking that statement seriously would force the reader to question the bumper sticker. It makes a flat, authoritative statement with the kind of "because I said so" authority that rubs most people the wrong way. How much wisdom and credibility do bumper stickers have? Practically none. Of *all* "authorities," they ought to be questioned!

But the truth is that most advertising and too much living are based on accepting authoritative statements that have no basis in reality. We're told we "deserve" breaks, deals, credit, perks, and any number of benefits attached to things we're being asked to buy. But we're not given a clear reason why we "deserve" these things. Some of the most treacherous, destructive, and irrational acts are committed by people who, when asked for a reason for their choices simply say, "I did it because I deserve to be happy." Granted, this may sound a little like one of the three inalienable rights identified in the Declaration of Independence, but that document claims we have a right to "pursue happiness," not a right to be happy. There's a huge difference.

This exposes a false philosophy of life confronted by Concept Four. Many of us believe in the ultimate law of our own comfort. We might not state it as briefly or crudely as the first bumper sticker, "If it feels good, do it," but that's exactly how we live. We're open to almost anything that holds out the hope of keeping us comfortable, pain free, and happy. How ironic that when we discover that living for our comfort doesn't produce the hoped for results, we simply redouble our efforts, instead of questioning the validity of our "philosophy." We need a better philosophy to live by. As Concept Four states, "In order to change, we have to replace our desire to comfort ourselves at all costs with a willingness to suffer just as Christ suffered for us."

The Bible passage for this session has to do with an exchange between some Greek strangers, Jesus' disciples, and Jesus. The Greeks and disciples approached Jesus for a conference; Jesus responded with a challenge. The newcomers wanted to meet Jesus. He responded by telling them what it would take to be His followers. This is one of the passages that gives LIFL its name. Jesus told His hearers that following Him meant *losing for life*. He said, "Those who love their life in this world will lose it. Those who care nothing for their life in this world will keep it for eternity" (John 12:25). Jesus didn't hesitate to tell anyone who would listen that some things in life are a lot more important than personal comfort and safety.

If those last sentences were easy to read, you may not have been paying attention. The statement Jesus made offended many of His listeners. People today may find them even more offensive. The idea of losing our life for the sake of anything is unacceptable to most. We want "selective losing." We would like to lose a little weight, lose a habit here or there, and lose some problems—but losing life? Jesus was either issuing the ultimate true challenge, or He was out of His mind!

Before we dismiss Jesus' words, two notes need to be added. First, He lived by them. He practiced what He preached. Second, countless others who have put His words into action have found them to be true. So His challenge is worth another look. Jesus was answering our deepest desire: *How do I truly keep life?* He pointed out that we have a choice—we can love our lives now for a brief time and lose them for eternity, or we can let go of our lives now but keep them for eternity. Keeping life now is like gripping water. The more tightly we grasp, the more we are aware of it slipping away. Losing life now means holding life with an open hand. It means declaring ourselves no longer in control. Keeping life means a constant quest for comfort and safety. Losing life means walking under Christ's lordship and accepting suffering as part of taking Jesus seriously. He suffered for us. We follow Him by living in a way that doesn't avoid suffering at any cost.

In Jesus' words and actions we find two crucial answers: the answer for our struggle with sin and failure and the answer for the way to live. Other concepts in LIFL will expand on this truth, but Concept Four has identified "what must be let go," which was referred to in Concept Three. If we're not willing to "replace our desire to comfort ourselves at all costs," we are still practicing "stubborn resistance." But if we are deciding each day to follow Jesus, even if suffering is part of the plan, we will be in the best place to experience the kinds of changes God wants to bring about in our lives.

DISCUSSION QUESTIONS ABOUT SCRIPTURE

❖ Why do you think the Greeks wanted to meet Jesus?

_____

_____

_____

_____

_____

_____

_____

_____

_____

_____

❖ Why would listeners be shocked by Jesus' statement about losing their lives?

_____

_____

_____

_____

_____

_____

_____

_____

_____

❖ What pain did Jesus endure during His life on earth?

_____

_____

_____

_____

_____

_____

_____

_____

_____

_____

❖ Why did Jesus go through all of that?

_____

_____

_____

_____

_____

_____

❖ What do some people do to maintain their comfort at all costs?

_____

_____

_____

_____

_____

_____

❖ Why does change involve pain?

_____

_____

_____

_____

_____

_____

❖ What sacrifices will your weight-loss goal entail?

_____

_____

_____

_____

_____

_____

CASE STUDY

JEFF

"It's easy. All I have to do is wear this belt for an hour a day and the inches will disappear around my waist. Plus, it was only $14.95 for the next four months! I saw it on TV," explained Jeff.

Rick looked at him skeptically. "Are you really sure it will work? I mean, you don't really have to do very much."

"That's the point!" exclaimed Jeff. "I can still be comfortable, eat what I want, and watch TV. In fact, I can watch TV while I wear the belt."

We may wonder why anyone could possibly believe that simply wearing a belt could melt away fat and pounds, but people keep falling for the ads and buying such worthless gadgets. This highlights the unfortunate truth that people want to accomplish difficult tasks as easily as possible; hence the numerous TV ads that promise quick weight loss with very little effort. The problem is, they never seem to work.

YOUR TURN

❖ Why did Jeff buy the belt device?

_____

_____

_____

_____

❖ Why don't these quick weight loss plans work?

_____

_____

_____

_____

❖ What other methods/techniques/products offer quick weight loss?

_____

_____

_____

_____

AS A GROUP

❖ Why are we so afraid to suffer?

_____

_____

_____

_____

_____

❖ How do we find ourselves looking for the "quick fix"?

_____

_____

_____

_____

_____

❖ In what areas of life do you try to keep comfortable and refuse to suffer?

_____

_____

_____

_____

_____

❖ What is the first step you need to take to get out of your comfort zone?

_____

_____

_____

_____

_____

CHALLENGE

Are you in a "keeping my life" mode—playing it safe and comfortable? If you really want to make progress, if you want to change, you will need to move out of that comfort zone and be willing to endure hardship and to sacrifice. With no pain, you'll have no gain!

DAILY DEVOTIONAL JOURNAL

DAY 1

Scripture: 1 PETER 4:1–2

So then, since Christ suffered physical pain, you must arm yourselves with the same attitude he had, and be ready to suffer, too. For if you have suffered physically for Christ, you have finished with sin. You won't spend the rest of your lives chasing your own desires, but you will be anxious to do the will of God.

DEVOTIONAL THOUGHT

Peter used the example of Christ's suffering to let the early Christians know that they would likely have to suffer as well. In other words, he is saying that suffering comes with the territory when you follow Jesus. This is not a cali to masochism but a challenge to approach life with the right attitude, a willingness to suffer if that's what it takes.

And notice the link between thinking right and living right. Anyone who has seriously decided to stop sinning and live God's way should be ready and willing to suffer. Don't let your desire to be comfortable keep you from God's best.

TRUTH I WILL FOCUS ON TODAY

_____

_____

_____

_____

MY PRAYER

_____

_____

_____

_____

DAY 2

Scripture: 1 JOHN 4:9–10

God showed how much he loved us by sending his one and only Son into the world so that we might have eternal life through him. This is real love—not that we loved God, but that he loved us and sent his Son as a sacrifice to take away our sins.

DEVOTIONAL THOUGHT

Our model for sacrificial living is Jesus Himself. He left heaven, became a human baby, lived in poverty under Roman rule, was falsely accused and convicted, was cursed, spat upon, beaten, and, finally, was crucified. Why? So that we might have life, eternal life. Now that's love!

So when you're feeling tired from the exercise, hungry from the diet, and desperate for the fatty foods you used to consume by the bucket, remember what He did for you. And push on!

TRUTH I WILL FOCUS ON TODAY

_____

_____

_____

_____

MY PRAYER

_____

_____

_____

_____

DAY 3

Scripture: 1 CORINTHIANS 9:24–27

Don't you realize that in a race everyone runs, but only one person gets the prize? So run to win! All athletes are disciplined in their training. They do it to win a prize that will fade away, but we do it for an eternal prize. So I run with purpose in every step. I am not just shadowboxing. I discipline my body like an athlete, training it to do what it should. Otherwise, I fear that after preaching to others I myself might be disqualified.

DEVOTIONAL THOUGHT

In this passage, the apostle Paul uses the athlete as an example of someone who exercises discipline and self-control to train for victory. Paul's point? A prize worth winning is worth sacrificing for.

Do *you* want victory? Is that your goal? What will it cost you in discipline and self-control?

TRUTH I WILL FOCUS ON TODAY

_____

_____

_____

_____

MY PRAYER

_____

_____

_____

_____

DAY 4

Scripture: PHILIPPIANS 3:13–14

No, dear brothers and sisters, I have not achieved it, but I focus on this one thing: Forgetting the past and looking forward to what lies ahead, I press on to reach the end of the race and receive the heavenly prize for which God, through Christ Jesus, is calling us.

DEVOTIONAL THOUGHT

Paul returns to the athletic image and compares his life to running a race, much like the marathon described previously in this session. Put yourself in the place of the runner who has about a mile to go in a marathon. Despite blisters, aches, cramps, and sharp pains in joints and lungs, the runner pushes through and pushes on, the goal in sight. Soon he or she will finish and receive the prize! The key is not to focus on the past or even the present discomfort, but to look forward to the finish and keep one's eyes on the goal.

What is your goal? What can you do to keep it in sight?

TRUTH I WILL FOCUS ON TODAY

_____

_____

_____

MY PRAYER

_____

_____

_____

_____

DAY 5

Scripture: 2 TIMOTHY 2:3–6

Endure suffering along with me, as a good soldier of Christ Jesus. Soldiers don't get tied up in the affairs of civilian life, for then they cannot please the officer who enlisted them. And athletes cannot win the prize unless they follow the rules. And hardworking farmers should be the first to enjoy the fruit of their labor.

DEVOTIONAL THOUGHT

Athletes aren't the only ones who suffer for a goal. Paul includes soldiers and farmers as examples. Today whom else might he include? Business people, teachers, police officers, parents? In fact, just about anyone who does well in his or her job succeeds through dedication and hard work.

Paul's point is that followers of Christ should expect to suffer and work hard if they are serious about their faith. But it also follows that you will need to "endure suffering" if you are serious about changing your lifestyle and developing healthy habits. Are you up to the challenge?

TRUTH I WILL FOCUS ON TODAY

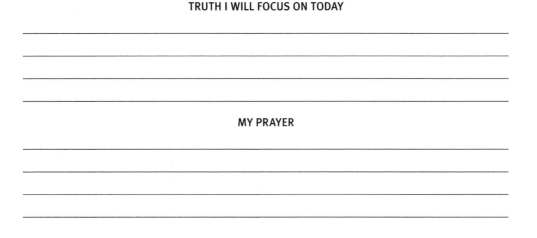

MY PRAYER

DAY 6

Scripture: ROMANS 12:1

And so, dear brothers and sisters, I plead with you to give your bodies to God because of all he has done for you. Let them be a living and holy sacrifice—the kind he will find acceptable. This is truly the way to worship him.

DEVOTIONAL THOUGHT

Before Christ came, pious Jews had to sacrifice animals to atone for their sins. But then Jesus came and became the ultimate, final blood sacrifice for sin. The old sacrificial system was finished. The Roman believers to whom Paul was writing these words knew the realities to which he was alluding.

But Paul says that believers themselves need to be living sacrifices. This means giving ourselves totally to our Lord—in effect, sacrificing our lives for His kingdom. Dead to sin, we become fully alive as we serve God.

Have you given your body to God? What does this imply for how you should live?

TRUTH I WILL FOCUS ON TODAY

_____

_____

_____

_____

MY PRAYER

_____

_____

_____

_____

DAY 7

Scripture: HEBREWS 12:1–4

Therefore, since we are surrounded by such a huge crowd of witnesses to the life of faith, let us strip off every weight that slows us down, especially the sin that so easily trips us up. And let us run with endurance the race God has set before us. We do this by keeping our eyes on Jesus, the champion who initiates and perfects our faith. Because of the joy awaiting him, he endured the cross, disregarding its shame. Now he is seated in the place of honor beside God's throne. Think of all the hostility he endured from sinful people; then you won't become weary and give up. After all, you have not yet given your lives in your struggle against sin.

DEVOTIONAL THOUGHT

Here the author of Hebrews picks up the racing metaphor and takes it a step further. He points out that in addition to focusing on the goal, the successful runner must shed anything that might slow the pace or impede his or her progress.

Often getting rid of those weights can be our most painful training exercise. These hindrances might include destructive relationships, harmful habits, or secret indulgences. But we need to get rid of them. We'll never get up to speed or make progress if we cling to them.

What "weight" do you need to "strip off" and let go of?

TRUTH I WILL FOCUS ON TODAY

_____

_____

_____

_____

MY PRAYER

_____

_____

_____

_____

Weekly Progress and Goals

❖ Current weight: _____

❖ Pounds lost this week: _____

NEW INSIGHTS

❖ About myself:

_____

_____

❖ From Scripture:

_____

_____

❖ About weight loss:

_____

_____

PLAN FOR NEXT WEEK

❖ Personal issue to focus on:

_____

_____

❖ Biblical truth to live out:

_____

_____

❖ Food to eliminate or restrict for the week:

_____

_____

❖ Exercise goals:

_____

_____

INTRODUCTION

All her life, Missy got whatever she wanted. As a child, her parents bought her every doll she saw and wanted. She had her ears pierced in elementary school. Entering junior high, she convinced her parents to allow her to wear makeup and begin the school year with a whole new wardrobe. On her sixteenth birthday, she received a brand new red Mazda Myata as a gift. No wonder that she threw a full-out tantrum during her senior year of high school, erupting at the principal, screaming and shouting about her rights and what she deserved.

That example may seem extreme, but entitlement has become a common attitude in our culture. There is a prevailing idea that we are entitled to certain rights and privileges, that we *deserve* them. We may even believe that *whatever* we do is correct and then excuse our bad behavior. After all, we deserve to have what we want, right? Wrong. God never promised us that life would be fair. He doesn't promise that we will be thin or never have to suffer or wait for anything. You are not the exception to the rule.

VIDEO 5

Notes from video:

_____

_____

_____

_____

_____

_____

_____

_____

_____

_____

_____

LIFL CONCEPT 5

ARROGANT ENTITLEMENT WILL LEAD TO A LIFE OF UNREALISTIC EXPECTATIONS AND UNHEALTHY CHOICES WHEN WHATEVER YOU BELIEVE YOU ARE ENTITLED TO IS MISSING FROM YOUR LIFE.

No one owes you anything. Just because you are intelligent doesn't mean you deserve an A+ and should get one automatically. Being nice to people doesn't insure they won't hurt you. Following God doesn't guarantee that you won't suffer. Getting a promotion doesn't allow you to celebrate and eat anything you want without gaining weight. Living a good life doesn't mean you deserve to be thin.

We may not want to admit it, but all people believe that they deserve *something*. That belief can keep us from enjoying life. For example, realizing that we didn't get everything on our wish list, we can overlook the gifts we *have* received. Or believing that we deserve a bigger house, we can fail to be thankful for having shelter. Or feeling that we deserve to eat whatever we want, we can forget that millions of starving people crave any food at all.

When do you feel that you deserve more, that you're entitled? How do you respond when events don't turn out as you envisioned? What can you do to make the change from entitlement to gratitude?

SCRIPTURE

LUKE 15:11–32

To illustrate the point further, Jesus told them this story: "A man had two sons. The younger son told his father, 'I want my share of your estate now before you die.' So his father agreed to divide his wealth between his sons.

"A few days later this younger son packed all his belongings and moved to a distant land, and there he wasted all his money in wild living. About the time his money ran out, a great famine swept over the land, and he began to starve. He persuaded a local farmer to hire him, and the man sent him into his fields to feed the pigs. The young man became so hungry that even the pods he was feeding the pigs looked good to him. But no one gave him anything.

"When he finally came to his senses, he said to himself. 'At home even the hired servants have food enough to spare, and here I am dying of hunger! I will go home to my father and say, "Father, I have sinned against both heaven and you, and I am no longer worthy of being called your son. Please take me on as a hired servant.'"

"So he returned home to his father. And while he was still a long way off, his father saw him coming. Filled with love and compassion, he ran to his son, embraced him, and kissed him. His son said to him, 'Father, I have sinned against both heaven and you, and I am no longer worthy of being called your son.'

"But his father said to the servants, 'Quick! Bring the finest robe in the house and put it on him. Get a ring for his finger and sandals for his feet. And kill the calf we have been fattening. We must celebrate with a feast, for this son of mine was dead and has now returned to life. He was lost, but now he is found.' So the party began.

"Meanwhile, the older son was in the fields working. When he returned home, he heard music and dancing in the house, and he asked one of the servants what was going on. 'Your brother is back,' he was told, 'and your father has killed the fattened calf. We are celebrating because of his safe return.'

"The older brother was angry and wouldn't go in. His father came out and begged him, but he replied, 'All these years I've slaved for you and never once refused to do a single thing you told me to. And in all that time you never gave me even one young goat for a feast with my friends. Yet when this son of yours comes back after squandering your money on prostitutes, you celebrate by killing the fattened calf!'

"His father said to him, 'Look, dear son, you have always stayed by me, and everything I have is yours. We had to celebrate this happy day. For your brother was dead and has come back to life! He was lost, but now he is found!'"

The story of the Prodigal Son is so familiar that we may have decided long ago that it doesn't apply to us. If we are not a younger son, a father, or an older brother, we may assume a spectator's place rather than a participant's role in the story. But Jesus' parable includes timeless human experiences that are repeated in every generation. Every person has been a child. We vaguely or vividly remember what we assumed our existence entitled us to receive. And many of us grew up thinking we were the center of the universe. But people and events eventually get around to letting us know the world doesn't actually revolve around us. This is not an easy or pleasant lesson to learn.

Early misconceptions die hard. Do our feelings of worthlessness flow from the discovery that we are not the center of the universe or from the pain caused by people who will not recognize us as such? Is the problem theirs or ours? Most would agree that every human being is entitled to basic dignity. But people seldom settle for dignity alone. We grasp for a lot more. We want what's fair but secretly strive for a larger piece of the pie. And our desires often veer into arrogant entitlement.

The young son in Jesus' parable was a poster child for arrogant entitlement. He took his upbringing and heritage for granted. He had trouble appreciating what he had because it had all come to him without any effort, sacrifice, or pain. Evidently the only area of pain in his short life was the frustration over not being able to live on his own. He took that as a birthright, along with the resources to make independent living a reality.

There's an uncomfortable familiarity in the young son's attitude when he tells his father, "I want my share of your estate now before you die." The easy assumption that certain things should just be, and the sooner the better, is the telltale sign of arrogant entitlement. And we sometimes express that attitude. Not only did the young son think he should get what was coming to him right then, he also took for granted that he would know what to do with it when he got it.

Unfortunately, a very large part of arrogance is actually ignorance. The young man's freedom and independence was an illusion. He was entirely dependent on what his father had given him, only now it was a resource with limits. And he didn't understand the meaning of limits of any kinds—appetites, relationships, and choices. The young son didn't recognize consequences and was blind to his dwindling supplies until he came up empty. Suddenly his money was gone, his friends had vanished, and his freedom had become severely limited. He ignored the hard realities of life until they smacked him in the face and he woke up in a pigsty.

Luke 15:17–19 shows us that this boy discovered the same truths as LIFL Concepts One through Five. Everything became painfully clear to him. Suddenly he realized he had exchanged a wonderful living for a lifestyle that couldn't last. The unrealistic expectations and unhealthy choices that were based on his arrogant entitlement became obvious in the harsh light of reality. The shock wiped away any stubborn resistance he might have been tempted to exercise. He was ready for the hope and humiliation of going home.

All this may seem like overkill. After all, we haven't gone *that* far in assuming that the world revolves around us! In fact, our reluctance to identify with the little brother may lead us to feel a little like the older brother. We don't seem to get away with half of what other people get away with! And people who have messed up their lives royally seem to gain such easy forgiveness. We haven't done anything all that bad—do we even need forgiveness? But note that the older brother went away in bitterness. He had his own brand of arrogant entitlement. He assumed he should be particularly rewarded for sticking around, but his response indicates his envy and anger toward his little brother. Until he got over his own stubborn resistance, he would have to remain in the prison and chains he had forged himself.

LIFL Concept Five measures a step of progress by taking a step back from life. All these concepts or principles represent choices. Each time we make a right choice, we get to move toward the benefits of the next concept. Each time we make a wrong choice, we experience the consequences of the next concept. The longer we ignore Concept Four and spend our resources on "comforting ourselves at all costs," the more we will become aware that things are "missing" from our lives. Sooner or later, as the younger son discovered, we will run out of resources. The means we arrogantly assumed would not end turn out to be limited. Waking up empty may turn out to be the best, or worst, moment of life. It becomes the worst when we exercise stubborn resistance and decide to live our way, even in the pigsty. It wasn't just where he was that awakened the young man; it was realizing that the pods the pigs ate were looking tasty. He couldn't remain in the pigsty and not become a pig.

But waking up can become the best moment when we make it a turning point—when we give up all entitlement and decide we'll return to the Father, the One who gave us everything we've wasted up to this point in life. At the moment we begin to leave the pigsty, Concept Five gives way to Concept Six.

DISCUSSION QUESTIONS ABOUT SCRIPTURE

❖ What choices did the younger son make?

_____

_____

_____

_____

_____

_____

_____

_____

❖ What was the turning point in the son's thinking?

_____

_____

_____

_____

_____

_____

_____

❖ How did the older brother respond to the younger brother's return?

_____

_____

_____

_____

_____

❖ Why did he respond that way?

_____

_____

_____

_____

_____

❖ In what ways are you like the younger son? The older son?

_____

_____

_____

_____

_____

_____

CASE STUDY

KATRINA

Life was going well for Katrina. She was succeeding in work and at home. Of course, with every success came a celebration. When she finished her big project at work, she went out to eat for a big dinner. When she got a promotion, there was plenty of cake to eat. When her son graduated from high school, she prepared a decadent dinner for the family to enjoy.

Sure, Katrina was trying to lose her "baby weight" from her last child (now eight years old), but she needed to celebrate. And all celebrations required food. With all of her hard work, she deserved to have some chocolate. *She* was the one who got the raise. It was *her* son who was a National Merit Scholar.

YOUR TURN

❖ What did Katrina feel was entitled to her?

_____

_____

_____

_____

_____

_____

❖ Why did she feel she deserved the reward?

_____

_____

_____

_____

_____

_____

❖ Why wasn't Katrina losing weight?

_____

_____

_____

_____

_____

_____

❖ In what ways does Katrina need to change?

_____

_____

_____

_____

_____

_____

AS A GROUP

❖ What do you feel that you "deserve"?

_____

_____

_____

_____

_____

❖ When do you feel most entitled?

_____

_____

_____

_____

_____

❖ How do _you_ need to change?

_____

_____

_____

_____

_____

CHALLENGE

Falling into the entitlement trap is easy because that attitude is so prevalent today. Advertisements tell us that we "are worth it" and encourage us to pamper ourselves because we "deserve it." We expect family, friends, neighbors, co-workers, and even the government to meet _our_ needs. No wonder making excuses comes easy to us and we find it difficult to take personal responsibility for our actions. But that outlook on life will only lead to unrealistic expectations and, ultimately, to disappointment and failure.

Don't go that way. Instead, thank God for the physical, mental, social, and spiritual resources He has given you, and take responsibility for your life.

DAILY DEVOTIONAL JOURNAL

DAY 1

Scripture: PROVERBS 14:16

The wise are cautious and avoid danger; fools plunge ahead with reckless confidence.

DEVOTIONAL THOUGHT

Confidence in itself isn't bad, and that's not what this verse is saying. Rather, the point here is that some people are so filled with themselves, so arrogant, that they do very foolish actions "with reckless confidence." Despite all the facts to the contrary, they believe they know best and plunge ahead.

Ask God to give you a healthy dose of His wisdom so that you'll know when to act and when to wait.

TRUTH I WILL FOCUS ON TODAY

_____

_____

_____

_____

MY PRAYER

_____

_____

_____

_____

DAY 2

Scripture: 1 CORINTHIANS 4:18–20

Some of you have become arrogant, thinking I will not visit you again. But I will come—and soon—if the Lord lets me, and then I'll find out whether these arrogant people just give pretentious speeches or whether they really have God's power. For the Kingdom of God is not just a lot of talk; it is living by God's power.

DEVOTIONAL THOUGHT

The church at Corinth had big problems, and Paul confronted them. As their spiritual mentor and friend and as a leader in the early Christian church, he felt responsible for them and he acted strongly to turn the church around. Obviously, one of Paul's main concerns was the arrogance of some people in the church. They talked big but were far from the truth, and they were pulling others down with them.

Pride and arrogance can blind us to the truth. That's when we need a "Paul" to confront us with our actions and keep us accountable. Who do you have in your life to tell you the uncomfortable truth about your choices and life direction?

TRUTH I WILL FOCUS ON TODAY

_____

_____

_____

_____

MY PRAYER

_____

_____

_____

_____

DAY 3

Scripture: PSALM 103:10

He does not punish us for all our sins; he does not deal harshly with us, as we deserve.

DEVOTIONAL THOUGHT

"I deserve it!" "I just want what's coming to me!" You've probably heard statements like that or have made them yourself. When someone less "deserving" gets the award; when someone's metabolism allows that person to eat virtually anything and not gain an ounce; when we are blamed for something we didn't do—we wonder at the injustice and focus on what *should* have happened.

But do we really want to get what we deserve? As this psalm reminds us, God has *not* judged us for all our sins—we "deserve" much worse that we are getting. Instead of thinking of all that you are entitled to, consider the countless gifts you've received from your loving Father—totally undeserved. It's all about His grace.

TRUTH I WILL FOCUS ON TODAY

_____

_____

_____

_____

MY PRAYER

_____

_____

_____

_____

DAY 4

Scripture: PROVERBS 25:27

It's not good to eat too much honey, and it's not good to seek honors for yourself.

DEVOTIONAL THOUGHT

Honey is sweet and nutritious—stir some in your tea or spread some on your toast. But imagine how you'd feel after downing a whole glass of the golden goo—pretty queasy. And that's the point of this proverb.

Receiving an honor can be like a taste of honey—so sweet. But obsessing about what we didn't get that we think we deserve can sour us quickly. So watch out for arrogant entitlement—it'll make you sick.

TRUTH I WILL FOCUS ON TODAY

_____

_____

_____

_____

MY PRAYER

_____

_____

_____

_____

DAY 5

Scripture: LUKE 6:32

If you love only those who love you, why should you get credit for that? Even sinners love those who love them!

DEVOTIONAL THOUGHT

Some people are so worried about being noticed and getting credit that they want to be praised for every action, even ones that take no sacrifice or effort. Again, this comes from a self-centered attitude that assumes the individual "deserves" this or that.

Instead of focusing on what you deserve or on getting praised for every good deed and positive step, keep your life in perspective. Measure yourself and your actions by God's standard and determine to live His way.

TRUTH I WILL FOCUS ON TODAY

_____

_____

_____

_____

MY PRAYER

_____

_____

_____

_____

DAY 6

Scripture: EPHESIANS 3:8

Though I am the least deserving of all God's people, he graciously gave me the privilege of telling the Gentiles about the endless treasures available to them in Christ.

DEVOTIONAL THOUGHT

Do you see the irony in this verse? Paul, the courageous, gifted, brilliant apostle and leader of the early church and the greatest Christian missionary of all time, says he is the least deserving Christian there is. And he considers the opportunity to tell others about Jesus to be an amazing privilege.

What a contrast to many people these days who think they deserve every accolade and perk. You'll make little progress in the Christian life, or life in general, with that attitude. Instead, take a realistic assessment of yourself and your situation, and ask God to guide you His way.

TRUTH I WILL FOCUS ON TODAY

_____

_____

_____

_____

MY PRAYER

_____

_____

_____

_____

DAY 7

Scripture: MATTHEW 16:24

Then Jesus said to his disciples, "If any of you wants to be my follower, you must turn from your selfish ways, take up your cross, and follow me."

DEVOTIONAL THOUGHT

When Jesus' disciples heard this statement, they knew what it meant to "take up a cross." They had seen Roman crucifixions, so they knew Jesus was calling them to be willing to die, spiritually speaking. Following Him would probably mean losing everything else. No self-centeredness allowed.

They did give up everything and chose to follow Jesus. In the process, they turned their backs on the world and on their own desires. For many others, however, selfish ambition kept them from following Jesus and His calling on their lives. And they missed the Savior.

Where are you when it comes to "selfish ways"? What keeps you from following Jesus fully?

TRUTH I WILL FOCUS ON TODAY

_____

_____

_____

_____

MY PRAYER

_____

_____

_____

_____

WEEKLY PROGRESS AND GOALS

❖ Current weight: _____

❖ Pounds lost this week: _____

NEW INSIGHTS

❖ About myself:

_____

_____

❖ From Scripture:

_____

_____

❖ About weight loss:

_____

_____

_____

PLAN FOR NEXT WEEK

❖ Personal issue to focus on:

_____

_____

❖ Biblical truth to live out:

_____

_____

❖ Food to eliminate or restrict for the week:

_____

_____

❖ Exercise goals:

_____

_____

INTRODUCTION

A woman decides to join a local health club. Motivated to do it right, she pays extra and hires a personal trainer. On the first day, her trainer assigns a variety of exercises. Instead of trying them, however, the woman complains that the exercises are too strenuous for her. Even with the trainer's urgings and encouragement, she refuses to budge. Taking a different approach, the trainer suggests an easier routine. Again the woman balks. Eventually the hour session ends with the woman doing virtually nothing.

As this scene is repeated each day, the woman loses no weight and becomes increasingly frustrated. She thinks, *This is the trainer's fault. The exercises are too difficult. I might hurt myself.* All of the trainer's knowledge means nothing to her. She isn't willing to submit and do the work.

This woman says she wants to change, to get in shape and lose weight. She's on the right train, but she won't let it run on the right tracks. What good things might happen if she could just humble herself a little bit, instead of rejecting her program outright?

VIDEO 6

Notes from video:

_____

_____

_____

_____

_____

_____

_____

_____

_____

_____

_____

LIFL CONCEPT 6

WHEN WE HUMBLE OURSELVES AND SURRENDER BEFORE GOD, WE BEGIN TO MAKE PROGRESS; AND WHEN WE DO THIS DAILY, WE MAINTAIN A HEALTHY LIFE, FREE OF BEHAVIORS THAT CONTROL US OR PEOPLE WHOM WE DESIRE TO CONTROL.

The biggest factor in many conflicts is wanting to control a situation or a person. Co-workers belittle each other to try to prove who is in control. We argue with people usually because we can't admit we are wrong and want our own way. With many addictions, too, it's all about control. People who are obsessive-compulsive try to control the world around them and keep things in place. Everyone wants to control someone or something. Perhaps we try to control others because we can't control ourselves.

In order to change your eating habits, you must surrender up to God all the people you are trying to control. As you submit those relationships to *His* control, it will give you the freedom to release your eating habits to Him as well. God knows everything about you and knows what is best for you. Surrender your problems to Him.

SCRIPTURE

EPHESIANS 4:17–32

With the Lord's authority I say this: Live no longer as the Gentiles do, for they are hopelessly confused. Their minds are full of darkness; they wander far from the life God gives because they have closed their minds and hardened their hearts against him. They have no sense of shame. They live for lustful pleasure and eagerly practice every kind of impurity.

But that isn't what you learned about Christ. Since you have heard about Jesus and have learned the truth that comes from him, throw off your old sinful nature and your former way of life, which is corrupted by lust and deception. Instead, let the Spirit renew your thoughts and attitudes. Put on your new nature, created to be like God—truly righteous and holy.

So stop telling lies. Let us tell our neighbors the truth, for we are all parts of the same body. And "don't sin by letting anger control you." Don't let the sun go down while you are still angry, for anger gives a foothold to the devil.

If you are a thief, quit stealing. Instead, use your hands for good hard work, and then give generously to others in need. Don't use foul or abusive language. Let everything you say be good and helpful, so that your words will be an encouragement to those who hear them.

And do not bring sorrow to God's Holy Spirit by the way you live. Remember, he has identified you as his own, guaranteeing that you will be saved on the day of redemption.

Get rid of all bitterness, rage, anger, harsh words, and slander, as well as all types of evil behavior. Instead, be kind to each other, tenderhearted, forgiving one another, just as God through Christ has forgiven you.

If we can picture life running as if it were on train tracks, then every person's existence would be going one of two directions. The first five LIFL concepts were all about recognizing that our train is headed the wrong way and that we need to make certain choices before the train gets turned around and headed in the right direction. The concept of repentance in the Bible describes this very picture of a life headed one way that makes a one-hundred-and-eighty-degree turn to head in the opposite direction. To use Jesus' words that we looked at in Concept Four, one way of life on the tracks leads to an eternal loss of life; the other way of life on the tracks leads to eternal life. Concept Six describes the turn. It identifies those moments when we stop heading the wrong way and begin heading the right way. It tells us what's involved in moving day-by-day in the right direction. When we "humble ourselves and surrender before God," we are releasing the controls of the train and stepping back. The LIFL concepts will now deal with the new experience of life headed in the direction of eternity with God. The way isn't easy, but it's right.

The apostle Paul had a special appreciation for the Christians in Ephesus. He had spent several years with them. Afterward, he wrote this short, power-packed letter to them, drawing the big picture and explaining many of the delightful details of the Christian life. Just as Concept Six marks a turning point in the LIFL approach, the fourth chapter of Ephesians signals a shift in Paul's words to his audience. The first three chapters of the letter are foundational. They help us see our value and identity in Christ as part of God's great plan. The next chapter begins with a "therefore"—a term that alerts us to an important decision. If what we've read in the first three chapters is true, then what we read in the next three chapters are applications that logically and spiritually follow.

Ephesians 4 is filled with practical guidelines for living "a life worthy of your calling" (Ephesians 4:1). The original language of this picture is "walk worthy"—make progress in the right direction. Once a life has been "turned around on the tracks," it's time to start moving in the right direction.

While we're thinking about life as train tracks, we might also consider the difference between *trying* to change and *training* to change. Most of us are experts in "trying." We may have tried to change some behavior so often that we've given up all hope. Why is this? Why does *trying to change* most often really mean *staying the same*? This is because "trying" has no way to handle failure. When we try and fail, we stop trying.

Training operates with a different mindset. It expects a certain amount of failure. Training sees the objective and makes deliberate steps toward it, even though no one step in the right direction spans the whole distance. The preparation for running a marathon involves constant failure. Those seriously training for a marathon are accomplishing various intermediary distances, but they never actually run a marathon to get ready for a marathon. You prepare for the long run by many shorter runs, not just by "trying" to run the whole thing once in a while.

Among the directions Paul included in Ephesians 4 is a pattern we can use to deal with life's challenges. These verses can serve as a training plan for change, with three components: "throw off," "let the Spirit renew," and "put on" (4:22–23). As we identify attitudes and habits that are expressions of our "old sinful nature and former way of life," we reject them—throw them off. We own up to them, then disown them. We recognize they may have sunk deep roots in us, so we depend on God's Spirit to renew and cleanse us from them and their effects. This becomes a deliberate spiritual process in our lives, not something we're trying to do in our strength. Then we identify the positive alternative that can replace the old habit or attitude and make that our purpose. In this way, we put on our "new nature created to be like God—truly righteous and holy."

Ephesians 4:25–32 summarizes five case studies, illustrating what it means to apply these components in the areas of lying, anger, stealing, foul language, and abusive behaviors. For example, if we identify a problem with anger, then we "throw off" the anger by first deciding we can't let anger control us. If anger is our autopilot setting, it gives a "foothold to the devil." We're actually yielding control to someone who wants to destroy us! The renewal and "putting on" comes as we present our anger to God and ask for His Spirit's control. We learn that anger can be expressed without it being in control. In fact, we put on our new nature in Christ when we refuse to harbor anger overnight but settle it before the sun goes down.

We begin to benefit from Concept Six when *we* stop trying to change ourselves and enroll in *God's* gym for training in change. We accept the fact that we will experience failures along the way. Our goal is not perfection but growth (more on this idea in a later session). In the meantime, we focus our attention on humbly submitting to God's training program to bring about His changes in our lives. This will keep us on the right tracks.

DISCUSSION QUESTIONS ABOUT SCRIPTURE

❖ What do you think Paul meant by living "a life worthy of your calling" (Ephesians 4:1)?

_____

_____

_____

_____

_____

_____

❖ What might an *un*worthy life look like?

_____

_____

_____

_____

_____

_____

❖ What's the difference between *trying* to change and *training* to change?

_____

_____

_____

_____

_____

_____

❖ What training plan does Paul present in Ephesians 4?

_____

_____

_____

_____

_____

_____

❖ What might you need to "throw off" from your "former way of life"? What will that involve?

_____

_____

_____

_____

_____

❖ What do you need to "put on"? How can you do that?

_____

_____

_____

_____

_____

❖ Why is this important to do?

_____

_____

_____

_____

_____

_____

CASE STUDY

RENARD

Renard wasn't a rookie. At thirty-two, he could still beat his sixteen-year-old nephew, Kenan, on the basketball court one-on-one. Sure, he'd picked up a few pounds. And sure, the pounds weren't exactly disappearing as quickly as they had when he was Kenan's age. But he knew what he was doing. He said as much to his wife Joleyn when she decided to wave pamphlets from the doctor's office at him. As if he needed advice on losing weight.

"For the past year you've been saying you're going to lose fifteen pounds," she said.

"Under control," he replied.

Joleyn's look was skeptical. She jabbed a finger at the pamphlet. "It says here that during a workout, you need to get your heart rate up to the target rate. Basketball doesn't quite cut—"

"I don't need that," he interrupted, waving a dismissive hand. "I know what I'm doing. Don't forget, I played basketball in high school."

"Maybe if you talk to the doctor—"

"I said it's all under control!"

YOUR TURN

❖ Why wasn't Renard open to his wife's advice?

_____

_____

_____

_____

❖ What makes him think he has his weight and life "under control"?

_____

_____

_____

_____

❖ What do you think Joleyn could try to get through to Renard?

_____

_____

_____

_____

❖ What can be the first step in Renard's "training" routine?

_____

_____

_____

_____

AS A GROUP

❖ Why might it be difficult to submit to a training routine?

_____

_____

_____

_____

_____

❖ Besides exercise, what can be included in an effective training program to help us "throw off" bad habits?

_____

_____

_____

_____

_____

❖ Humbling ourselves and surrendering to God seem to be hard to do. Why is that?

_____

_____

_____

_____

_____

CHALLENGE

The idea of "trying" to change implies that we'll make a concerted effort to act differently when a tempting situation arises. However, "training" involves a conscious, thought out, step-by-step program of moving in the right direction. Training begins with a decision, a choice, and involves daily choices to do what has been decided.

God's gym for training in change is open. Walk through the door and enroll. Then humbly submit to His direction. Get started!

DAILY DEVOTIONAL JOURNAL

DAY 1

Scripture: PSALM 25:9

He leads the humble in doing what is right, teaching them his way.

DEVOTIONAL THOUGHT

Ever have trouble asking for directions? Many of us rationalize away our need for help, even when we're totally lost. "I don't need help. I can get there on my own." But can we? If we examine our past mistakes, the answer is no. Admitting that we need direction takes humility and teachability. God offers direction but does not force His people to take it.

In what ways do you sense God is leading you? What has He taught you about Himself in the past? Are you willing to go where He leads?

TRUTH I WILL FOCUS ON TODAY

_____

_____

_____

_____

MY PRAYER

_____

_____

_____

_____

DAY 2

Scripture: PROVERBS 3:34

The LORD mocks the mockers but is gracious to the humble.

DEVOTIONAL THOUGHT

In our society, we value talk show hosts and other celebrities who are quick with a sarcastic quip. We consider their targets deserving of these caustic comments. "Ha! Good one!" we cry. But how many of us would place the Lord in the category of the mocker? We can't picture Him sitting on the sidelines calling out comments like a theater heckler. But the message here is the absolute foolishness of pride. God sees through pride and scorns it. The humble, however, always have His full attention.

Humbly ask the Lord to show you areas in your life where pride might lurk. Be open to changing whatever He shows you.

TRUTH I WILL FOCUS ON TODAY

_____

_____

_____

_____

MY PRAYER

_____

_____

_____

_____

DAY 3

Scripture: 2 CHRONICLES 7:14

Then if my people who are called by my name will humble themselves and pray and seek my face and turn from their wicked ways, I will hear from heaven and will forgive their sins and restore their land.

DEVOTIONAL THOUGHT

Picture a field of sunflowers waving in the wind, their heads facing the east toward the rising sun. The sunflower constantly turns its face toward the sun, following the sun in its fiery path across the sky. They clearly need the sun for survival.

The verse above, one of the most quoted verses in the Bible, is a picture of humility. It gives the picture of a face constantly turned toward God and hands lifted in supplication. As a child of the Son, do you seek His face when the need arises? Do you soak in His rays of direction and take your nourishment from His Word?

TRUTH I WILL FOCUS ON TODAY

_____

_____

_____

_____

MY PRAYER

_____

_____

_____

_____

DAY 4

Scripture: 2 CHRONICLES 30:8

Do not be stubborn, as they were, but submit yourselves to the LORD. Come to his Temple which he has set apart as holy forever. Worship the LORD your God so that his fierce anger will turn away from you.

DEVOTIONAL THOUGHT

What comes to your mind when you read the word *stubborn*? A donkey who won't budge? The Israelites who wouldn't obey? Someone you know who clings to a destructive habit? We readily know when others are stubborn. We, too, can stubbornly cling to our agendas and attitudes, considering ourselves in the right. But God has a way of peeling back the carpets of the heart and revealing the hidden dust of wrong motives.

God warned the Israelites to avoid going on as they were. Doing so would have led to their destruction. Do you sense the Spirit's gentle reminder of an attitude or motive to which you might be clinging? His reminders come through people or circumstances. Take time today to pray about those gentle nudges.

TRUTH I WILL FOCUS ON TODAY

_____

_____

_____

_____

MY PRAYER

_____

_____

_____

_____

DAY 5

Scripture: HEBREWS 12:9

Since we respected our earthly fathers who disciplined us, shouldn't we submit even more to the discipline of the Father of our spirits, and live forever?

DEVOTIONAL THOUGHT

As teenagers our hackles would go up at times when someone (mainly a parent) told us what to do or corrected us. We were exploring our independence and thought we were getting it right. Or, we were embarrassed about blowing it. As adults, our hackles still may go up when the subject of discipline comes up. It's hard to be reminded of what we aren't doing and be corrected accordingly. But why is it so hard? Could pride be the culprit?

Our heavenly Parent disciplines His children as any loving parent does. He wants our trust and submission, rather than our justification or complaints about correction. How can you cheerfully submit this week?

TRUTH I WILL FOCUS ON TODAY

_____

_____

_____

_____

MY PRAYER

_____

_____

_____

_____

DAY 6

Scripture: LUKE 9:23

Then [Jesus] said to the crowd, "If any of you wants to be my follower, you must turn from your selfish ways, take up your cross daily, and follow me."

DEVOTIONAL THOUGHT

We can look at a magazine article or watch celebrities on news shows and easily point out the perceived vain ambitions of others. They seem to stand out like sore thumbs. But the "selfish ways" of our own hearts are not so easily discerned at times.

Jesus' words are the rubber-meets-the-road statement of the Christian faith. Daily we are called to lay aside pride and follow Jesus. So, what are these selfish ways to which Jesus refers? Any ambitions that take God out of the equation. Only you and God know what those are in your life. Why not meet with Him today in prayer and find out if any selfishness lurks in your life.

TRUTH I WILL FOCUS ON TODAY

_____

_____

_____

_____

MY PRAYER

_____

_____

_____

_____

DAY 7

Scripture: LUKE 11:3

Give us each day the food we need.

DEVOTIONAL THOUGHT

Daily we toil at a job, confident in our own strength and abilities. We may know where our next paycheck or meal is coming from, or think we do. But the prayer Jesus taught His disciples to pray acknowledges that God is the true source.

We often mouth the words, "Give us each day the food we need," without thinking deeply about them. Jesus, our Savior, reminded Satan that man does not live by bread alone but by every word that comes from God (Matthew 4:4). He modeled a life of dependence on God. He didn't make a move without checking with the Father first. Is that your daily habit?

TRUTH I WILL FOCUS ON TODAY

_____

_____

_____

_____

MY PRAYER

_____

_____

_____

_____

WEEKLY PROGRESS AND GOALS

❖ Current weight: _____

❖ Pounds lost this week: _____

NEW INSIGHTS

❖ About myself:

_____

_____

❖ From Scripture:

_____

_____

❖ About weight loss:

_____

_____

_____

PLAN FOR NEXT WEEK

❖ Personal issue to focus on:

_____

_____

❖ Biblical truth to live out:

_____

_____

❖ Food to eliminate or restrict for the week:

_____

_____

❖ Exercise goals:

_____

_____

INTRODUCTION

In the movie *Pay It Forward*, a social studies teacher gives his class the assignment of making a difference in the world. As a result, one boy decides to "pay it forward" instead of *payback*. He believes that the world would be a better place if everyone just tried to help out a stranger, with no prospect of getting anything in return. Then that person would, in turn, help another stranger, and so it would continue. So the student "pays it forward" to three different people, and watches as they respond to help others.

Actually, that's how everyone should live. We all are connected and our actions directly and indirectly affect other people. Paying it forward requires humility and patience. One has to put the other person's needs ahead of his or her own.

You are not on your weight-loss journey alone. You are connected to others who are reaching for the same goal as you. Consider how you might be able to pay it forward to them today.

VIDEO 7

Notes from video:

_____

_____

_____

_____

_____

_____

_____

_____

_____

_____

_____

LIFL CONCEPT 7

CHRIST SET THE EXAMPLE OF HOW WE ARE TO HUMBLY SERVE EACH OTHER. IN HUMBLE SERVICE TO EACH OTHER WE STAY CONNECTED TO EACH OTHER AND TO CHRIST, WHO SET THE EXAMPLE WITH HIS LIFE.

As we learned in the last session, humbly submitting to someone else can be very difficult. That's because we want to control our lives as much as possible. Giving up that control is tough, but it's necessary—especially daily surrendering to God—if we want to progress in losing it for life.

The way of humility leads to thinking of others and serving them. Let's face it—we need others to help us along the way. And conversely, they need us. So we need to look for ways to connect with people whom we serve.

The greatest example of selfless service is none other than Jesus Christ. His life was all about serving. He served the crowds, His disciples, and ultimately, all of us, through His death on the cross. Follow your leader!

SCRIPTURE

JOHN 13:1–17

Before the Passover celebration, Jesus knew that his hour had come to leave this world and return to his Father. He had loved his disciples during his ministry on earth, and now he loved them to the very end. It was time for supper, and the devil had already prompted Judas, son of Simon Iscariot, to betray Jesus. Jesus knew that the Father had given him authority over everything and that he had come from God and would return to God. So he got up from the table, took off his robe, wrapped a towel around his waist, and poured water into a basin. Then he began to wash the disciples' feet, drying them with the towel he had around him.

When Jesus came to Simon Peter, Peter said to him, "Lord, are you going to wash my feet?"

Jesus replied, "You don't understand now what I am doing, but someday you will."

"No," Peter protested, "you will never ever wash my feet!"

> Jesus replied, "Unless I wash you, you won't belong to me."
>
> Simon Peter exclaimed, "Then wash my hands and head as well, Lord, not just my feet!"
>
> Jesus replied, "A person who has bathed all over does not need to wash, except for the feet, to be entirely clean. And you disciples are clean, but not all of you." For Jesus knew who would betray him. That is what he meant when he said, "Not all of you are clean."
>
> After washing their feet, he put on his robe again and sat down and asked, "Do you understand what I was doing? You call me 'Teacher' and 'Lord,' and you are right, because that's what I am. And since I, your Lord and Teacher, have washed your feet, you ought to wash each other's feet. I have given you an example to follow. Do as I have done to you. I tell you the truth, slaves are not greater than their master. Nor is the messenger more important than the one who sends the message. Now that you know these things, God will bless you for doing them."

Perhaps Jesus smiled as He rose from the table, wrapped the towel around His waist, and picked up the large bowl of water. He knew them so very well and yet loved them anyway. He knelt by one of His disciples and began to wash his feet. The faint odor of mud rose to compete with the succulent smells of the prepared food. The act of humility stunned them all. "What are we thinking?" they thought. "He shouldn't be doing *that*!" Still, it's telling that none of them rose to relieve Jesus of the duty. They all concluded, *Someone else should do that*. None of them thought, *I will do that*. Even Peter didn't volunteer to return the favor or take over the job. Ashamed and flustered, he simply declared, "You will never wash my feet!"

Jesus had to do this because His disciples (and we) would not have gotten the point otherwise. Service is not only the great equalizer; it is also the magnifying lens that reveals true leadership. No one is so great that he or she is exempt from serving, and no one is so insignificant that she or he is exempt from being served. It doesn't matter where we see ourselves on the shifting continuum of human importance; each of us *has been served!* God demonstrated loving service by giving His Son to the world (John 3:16). He came despite our universal equality as sinners undeserving of His love.

As Romans 5:6–8 states, "When we were utterly helpless, Christ came at just the right time and died for us sinners. Now, most people would not be willing to die for an upright person, though someone might perhaps be willing to die for a person who is especially good. But God showed his great love for us by sending Christ to die for us while we were still sinners." If no one else ever offered us a helping hand we would already be the recipients of the greatest act of service—someone has died for us!

In explaining His actions, Jesus made it clear that He was not compelled to wash His disciples' feet out of social pressure or necessity. He was, by their own words, their master and teacher. Yet He did the unexpected as an expression of love. And He added the following pointed application: "I have given you an example to follow. Do as I have done to you" (John 13:15).

Lord, lover, and leader—Jesus is all three to us. As Lord God incarnate, He deserves our worship and obedience. As God our friend and lover, He deserves our gratitude and responding love. As God our leader who gave us an example to follow, He deserves our painstaking loyalty. And He has asked us to imitate Him by serving others.

Most of us approach the LIFL program out of personal motivation. We are sensitive to our personal faults and failures. We think we have problems that need fixing. We may have even concluded that *we* are a problem that needs fixing. And we're right. We discover immediately through Concept One that we have to acknowledge responsibility for whatever prison of problems surrounds us. One of the truths that dawns on us as we grapple with Concept Two is that the truth we need must ultimately come from outside ourselves. Our problems aren't going to be solved by fresh insight. We need a more radical liberation. Someone must liberate us. Concepts Three through Six reveal what liberation will cost us, even though the price we pay doesn't buy us freedom. Someone else paid that price—Jesus Christ. We simply have to accept that freedom and let Jesus turn our train around on the tracks of life.

Along our way through the Concepts, other people have come into the picture. Applying Concept Six is impossible without involving others. The training routine we learned involves the people who populate our lives. Our LIFL experience begins with profound inward discoveries and challenges, but it quickly moves toward our external world. The internal transformation that God wants to bring about in us will be seen most clearly in the changes that come about in how we relate to others. Any definition of following Jesus that does not include serving others is hollow. Some of those whom we can serve are fellow participants in LIFL that we can encourage and help along the way. But the ones we serve will mostly be people who have little idea of what's happening to us as we apply the LIFL Concepts to living. They will probably be the first to notice that we are changing. It may start with questions about the fact that we're somehow acting differently.

We need to remember that longstanding patterns and habits that we found painful to break have impacted others. They may have gotten used to us being a certain negative way, so their first reaction to changes in us may be discomfort rather than delight. It will be normal for them to suspect the change to be temporary—that we will soon return to the way we've always acted. And if they ask, we should be quick to acknowledge their suspicions. It's more truthful to say, "Wow, I'm glad you've noticed a change. I'm not sure where this is going, and I realize I'll probably have some inconsistencies as we go, but I'm learning some concepts that are making a difference." We don't want to say, "I've completely changed. You can count on me for perfect behavior from now on." Those statements set them up for disappointment and set us up for failure.

The test of Concept Seven isn't whether others notice but whether or not we find ways to serve them as we follow Jesus Christ. We're not responsible for how others respond; we *are* responsible for our responses and obedience to Christ.

DISCUSSION QUESTIONS ABOUT SCRIPTURE

❖ Why were the disciples shocked that Jesus would stoop to wash their feet?

_____

_____

_____

_____

_____

❖ How did they respond?

_____

_____

_____

_____

_____

❖ How *didn't* they respond?

_____

_____

_____

_____

_____

❖ What reason did Jesus give for why He was doing this?

_____

_____

_____

_____

_____

❖ What does it mean for someone to call Jesus "Teacher and Lord"?

_____

_____

_____

_____

_____

❖ What does that mean for you? Whom do you need to serve?

_____

_____

_____

_____

_____

❖ In what other ways is Jesus your model?

_____

_____

_____

_____

_____

_____

CASE STUDY

KATHLEEN

Kathleen stopped herself from sighing loudly. Once again her friend Stacie was slowing her down. This was supposed to be an aerobic walk, not an aerobic crawl. They both had the same amount of weight to lose. Yet Stacie didn't seem as into weight-loss activities as much as Kathleen.

And no wonder, Kathleen thought. *She's been cheating on her diet.*

She knew that Stacie was a nervous eater. She ate when she felt out of control. And that seemed to be all the time lately since her divorce.

She needs more discipline in her life, Kathleen reasoned. *At work, at home, and especially over those kids who drive her crazy. And she was late again for our walk.*

"I'm ready to quit now," Stacie huffed, as she headed for the nearest park bench. "I don't know how you can keep up this pace."

"You've got to be disciplined about it, girl," Kathleen admonished. "You'll never lose the weight if you don't keep exercising."

As Stacie's countenance sagged with the rest of her body, Kathleen tried not to notice. What she said was for Stacie's own good, wasn't it? Nagging her was the only way to get her to keep to the goal.

YOUR TURN

❖ Why was Kathleen frustrated?

_____

_____

_____

_____

_____

_____

❖ What was Stacie's problem?

_____

_____

_____

_____

_____

❖ What might Kathleen do to help Stacie, to serve her?

_____

_____

_____

_____

_____

AS A GROUP

❖ Why do we need to connect with others in this LIFL process?

_____

_____

_____

_____

_____

❖ In what ways are family and friends helping you?

_____

_____

_____

_____

_____

❖ What might individuals be able to do to serve others who are in this program?

_____

_____

_____

_____

_____

_____

CHALLENGE

Jesus couldn't have been more clear in His interaction with the disciples in the Upper Room through His example and His words: He expected His disciples to wash feet, to humbly serve others, regardless of their title, status, or position in life. And remember, Jesus did and said this just before performing the ultimate act of service, submitting to the Cross, giving His life as a sacrifice for our sins.

Serving is often costly and inconvenient. But it's obedience to our Lord. And just as much as we need to be connected to others, to be served, they need us.

What can you do to help a family member, friend, co-worker, or neighbor _today_ who is also working hard to lose it for life?

DAILY DEVOTIONAL JOURNAL

DAY 1

Scripture: 1 JOHN 4:10

This is real love—not that we loved God, but that he loved us and sent his Son as a sacrifice to take away our sins.

DEVOTIONAL THOUGHT

We hand each other valentines and "I-love-you" messages on Sweetest Day or Valentine's Day and call it love. But God's example of love blows away any earthly attempts at showing love. Real love is allowing a Son to die for the wrongs He didn't commit. Real humility is knowing our need and accepting that love.

Real love is going out of your way to serve someone. Real humility is accepting whatever assignment God gives you to serve someone. In what tangible ways can you show real love to someone this week?

TRUTH I WILL FOCUS ON TODAY

_____

_____

_____

_____

MY PRAYER

_____

_____

_____

_____

DAY 2

Scripture: ROMANS 5:6–8

When we were utterly helpless, Christ came at just the right time and died for us sinners. Now, most people would not be willing to die for an upright person, though someone might perhaps be willing to die for a person who is especially good. But God showed his great love for us by sending Christ to die for us while we were still sinners.

DEVOTIONAL THOUGHT

When you were a baby, you couldn't do anything for yourself. A parent had to pick you up, feed you, dress you, and put you to bed. You could do nothing on your own except cry.

This passage reminds us that we're still helpless, even as adults. Our propensity to do wrong things makes us helpless. We need an intermediary—someone to make things right with God for us. But the good news is that Jesus willingly died for our wrongs. He didn't leave us as helpless as infants. How can you share this good news with others?

TRUTH I WILL FOCUS ON TODAY

_____

_____

_____

_____

MY PRAYER

_____

_____

_____

_____

DAY 3

Scripture: MICAH 6:8

No, O people, the LORD has told you what is good, and this is what he requires of you: to do what is right, to love mercy, and to walk humbly with your God.

DEVOTIONAL THOUGHT

Sometimes we want to assert to others that we know what's best. That's why we nag our children or our spouses and friends to do what's right. But sometimes, the best way to help is to be an example of humility, as the Lord used Micah to announce.

Perhaps instead of providing someone with yet another spoonful of well-meaning advice, we can pause and ask the Lord what's really needed in the situation. Maybe a listening ear? A quiet word of affirmation? A hug? How can you "do what is right" and show your love of mercy?

TRUTH I WILL FOCUS ON TODAY

_____

_____

_____

_____

MY PRAYER

_____

_____

_____

_____

DAY 4

Scripture: ROMANS 13:8–10

Owe nothing to anyone—except for your obligation to love one another. If you love your neighbor, you will fulfill the requirements of God's law. For the commandments say, "You must not commit adultery. You must not murder. You must not steal. You must not covet." These—and other such commandments—are summed up in this one commandment: "Love your neighbor as yourself." Love does no wrong to others, so love fulfills the requirements of God's law.

DEVOTIONAL THOUGHT

Many of us like to live debt free. We don't like credit card debt or overdrawn checking accounts. We also like to live debt free in relationships. "Keep a clean slate" is our motto. That's why we carefully give Christmas and birthday gifts to those who give us gifts. But as Paul writes in this passage, there are some debts we'll always have. We will always owe each other love.

What keeps this debt from being onerous is the fact that God loves people through us. We are truly His hands and feet. "I can do everything through Christ, who gives me strength" (Philippians 4:13). How will you pay your debt of love to someone today?

TRUTH I WILL FOCUS ON TODAY

_____

_____

_____

_____

MY PRAYER

_____

_____

_____

_____

DAY 5

Scripture: MATTHEW 7:12

Do to others whatever you would like them to do to you. This is the essence of all that is taught in the law and the prophets.

DEVOTIONAL THOUGHT

We call this verse the Golden Rule. Many of us learned it when we were kids. It is one rule that we would like other people to memorize in regard to us! We may quote it glibly as a reminder of what we're due. But like many of the statements of Jesus, this sentiment comes with a cost. Doing good to others may cost you time, tears, and a sacrifice of pride.

What do you expect others to do for you? Love you? Understand you? Be loyal to you? What are you willing to do for them?

TRUTH I WILL FOCUS ON TODAY

_____

_____

_____

_____

MY PRAYER

_____

_____

_____

_____

DAY 6

Scripture: **1 CORINTHIANS 12:4–7**

There are different kinds of spiritual gifts, but the same Spirit is the source of them all. There are different kinds of service, but we serve the same Lord. God works in different ways, but it is the same God who does the work in all of us. A spiritual gift is given to each of us so we can help each other.

DEVOTIONAL THOUGHT

What's your spiritual gift? We take tests and ask each other questions to confirm our gifting. After all, we want to be sure we're serving God "right." And sadly, we sometimes compare our gifts with others. "I wish I had Dave's gift of preaching." "I wish I could teach like Betsy." "I wish I could sing like Dana."

Each gift is under God's supreme control. The gifts are reminders that we're all in this together. One gift is no better than the other. Just as the body works together to function, so do we as believers. Even though you may be a "spleen" or a "colon," you're still part of the body! How will you use your gift(s) to serve others?

TRUTH I WILL FOCUS ON TODAY

_____

_____

_____

_____

MY PRAYER

_____

_____

_____

_____

DAY 7

Scripture: **PHILIPPIANS 2:16–18**

Hold firmly to the word of life; then, on the day of Christ's return, I will be proud that I did not run the race in vain and that my work was not useless. But I will rejoice even if I lose my life, pouring it out like a liquid offering to God, just like your faithful service is an offering to God. And I want all of you to share that joy. Yes, you should rejoice, and I will share your joy.

DEVOTIONAL THOUGHT

The little boy loved his first day of kindergarten and came home quite happy. When his mother woke him up for the second day of school, he said, "I have to go to school again? But I went yesterday." Sometimes we can fall into the same way of thinking as adults. "You mean I have to keep loving so and so?" (Fill in the name of a difficult person in your life.) But as Paul stated, "Even if I lose my life, pouring it out like a liquid offering." In other words, "Even if every ounce of my strength is used up to help you get to God, I'm willing to do whatever it takes." Are you?

TRUTH I WILL FOCUS ON TODAY

_____

_____

_____

_____

MY PRAYER

_____

_____

_____

_____

WEEKLY PROGRESS AND GOALS

❖ Current weight: _____

❖ Pounds lost this week: _____

NEW INSIGHTS

❖ About myself:

_____

_____

❖ From Scripture:

_____

_____

❖ About weight loss:

_____

_____

PLAN FOR NEXT WEEK

❖ Personal issue to focus on:

_____

_____

❖ Biblical truth to live out:

_____

_____

❖ Food to eliminate or restrict for the week:

_____

_____

❖ Exercise goals:

_____

_____

INTRODUCTION

In the Disney classic *Sleeping Beauty*, Princess Aurora's fairy godmothers decide to make a cake for her birthday. They aren't allowed to use their magic, so they decide to mix one from scratch. How hard could it be? Sure, they've never done this before, but it can't be *that* difficult, right? The picture makes it look so easy.

Numerous hours and bags of flour later, their masterpiece is complete. Except it's not beautiful or tasty looking at all. The layers are smashed and leaning different directions, and the icing is dripping onto the table. That's when the godmothers realize the difficulty of the task and resort to magic. And with a quick wave of a wand the four-layer cake is finished.

Wouldn't it be great to be able to wave a wand and transform a blob of butter, eggs, sugar and flour into a consummate culinary confection? To change cheap, drab clothes into designer apparel? To turn a bad day into a great one? Unfortunately, those shortcuts aren't available. We can't magically make our extra pounds go away or have problems disappear. We shouldn't expect change to occur instantly. Looking at pictures of famous people and their amazing weight loss doesn't mean that we will look the same way or have the same results.

Are you looking for a magic solution? Don't build your future on an illusion. Look to God for His recipe for contentment.

VIDEO 8

Notes from video:

_____

_____

_____

_____

_____

_____

_____

_____

_____

_____

LIFL CONCEPT 8

IN BETWEEN EXPECTATIONS AND REALITY IS MISERY, SO WE MUST ALWAYS BE EXAMINING OUR EXPECTATIONS IN ORDER TO EXPERIENCE SERENITY AND CONTENTMENT.

When the gap between the ideal and real is more like a chasm, we are susceptible to disappointment, discouragement, and even despair. This is true in many areas of life: career, finances, relationships, . . . and body image. Daily, cleverly designed and alluring advertisements, entertaining and intriguing TV shows and films, and other cultural media strongly imply that those goals are possible, reachable. And we'll always want more; we'll never have enough. Even when we try our hardest, our lives reflect a much different reality than those enticing images.

It's natural, of course, to dream of looking like a model, working at a satisfying and fulfilling (and extremely high paying) job, gaining money and possessions by the barn full, and enjoying conflict-free relationships. But attaining even one of those goals is highly unlikely. And if we've come to expect results like that, we may give up entirely.

The answer is not to set our sights so low that our goals mean nothing, even through they're reachable. That would be another type of self-deception. Instead, we need to take an honest assessment of where we are and get a reasonable idea of where we want to be. And then we need to decide what is really "enough."

Reexamine your expectations and see if they're realistic and attainable.

SCRIPTURE

1 TIMOTHY 6:6–10

Yet true godliness with contentment is itself great wealth. After all, we brought nothing with us when we came into the world, and we can't take anything with us when we leave it. So if we have enough food and clothing, let us be content.

But people who long to be rich fall into temptation and are trapped by many foolish and harmful desires that plunge them into ruin and destruction. For the love of money is the root of all kinds of evil. And some people, craving money, have wandered from the true faith and pierced themselves with many sorrows.

Certain advertisers want us to know how to spell "r-e-l-i-e-f" with their product. This kind of relief has the upside of being instantaneous and the downside of being only temporary, whereas *contentment* represents a larger and longer view of life. Faced with a choice between relief and contentment, contentment is the wiser option. This word puts a verbal finger on one of our deepest longings. We want to be content, even if we're not sure what it will take to achieve. When he was wrapping up his letter to Timothy, Paul gave some final counsel on the contents of contentment: "So if we have enough food and clothing, let us be content."

"Enough food and clothing," he said. Our understanding of contentment has a lot to do with our understanding of that term "enough." Many of us struggle to put any limits on our desires for feelings, food, and possessions. Our contentment depends on having enough of certain things, and when we have enough of that, then we think we will be content (satisfied, joy-filled, at peace). But if we need enough of something *before* we can be content, then we've defined our way into a prison of discontent. LIFL Concept One comes back to haunt us. If we feel chained by unbreakable discontent, we forged the links.

"Enough" is either a discovery or a decision. Those who approach having enough as a discovery think, *I don't know what enough of a particular thing is, but I'll know it when I see/feel/get it.* Unfortunately, trying to discover "enough" is like discovering the fountain of youth—it's nice to dream about, but the discovery never happens. We can't discover "enough" any more than we can discover the highest possible number—because whatever that number is, we can always add 1. Trying to discover how much food or drink is enough leads not to satisfaction but to sickness and stupor.

Finding the meaning of "enough" can also be a decision. We can decide what enough is for us. Our appetites don't have to have the last word, something they find impossible to utter. We can *tell* our appetites what will be enough. Making "enough" decisions doesn't mean we immediately have or will get enough, but it does mean we have a specific target. Deciding what enough is doesn't mean we can't accept or enjoy more than enough, but it creates a limitation on desires that otherwise refuse to be satisfied. Deciding what is enough opens the door to contentment.

Since most of us are in the habit of letting our appetites determine "enough," the idea of our having to decide what's enough can make us panic. Fortunately, our journey through the LIFL Concepts has included an introduction to the helper God has provided for us, His Holy Spirit. While "enough" remains a decision, it is not a decision we have to make entirely on our own and without any help. In deciding what enough is, we can also enlist the help of others who have experience in particular areas.

Along with God's Spirit and other people, we also have God's Word where we can find plenty of guidelines for deciding what is enough. The key passage for this session makes a good starting point. Paul writes, "Yet true godliness with contentment is itself great wealth" (1 Timothy 6:6). Then he points out the relative importance of the things we accumulate and worry about in this life before he turns to the objective again, "So if we have enough food and clothing, let us be content" (6:8). Being immortal, we're not going to take anything from this life that isn't also immortal. Qualities like godliness and contentment prepare us for eternity. Traits like greed and the love of money see no further than this life and lead to misery, uncertainty, and discontent.

LIFL Concept Eight states: "In between expectations and reality is misery, so we must always be examining our expectations in order to experience serenity and contentment." Trying to discover or decide what is enough can leave us open to the influences and pressures of the world. We need to always reexamine our thinking about "enough." This is because our tendency as humans is to drift into greed and discontent. Instead of expecting enough, we gradually want "more than enough."

Returning to our Scripture passage, what does godliness have to do with deciding about what's enough? The godly view of life has a deep trust in God's care and provision. Contentment realizes that feelings, appetites, and needs come and go, but God's character and purposes remain unchanged. God wants the best for us, no matter what we're experiencing at the moment. Our desires don't get the last word—God does. At any moment, God makes it possible for us to be content. If we have to add something to God in order to be content, then we don't yet understand contentment.

When writing Timothy, Paul used the temptation of money to illustrate the way our desires struggle with the wisdom of deciding what's enough. The descriptive words he uses in verses 9–10 ("long," "foolish and harmful desires," "love of money," and "craving") certainly apply not only to money but also to what money buys. Paul is warning that once we allow our desires to lead the way, not only will they not be satisfied, but they will also take us where we don't want to go. The last two phrases in verse 10 summarize all the sorrow created by a life lived outside the LIFL Concepts—a person who has "wandered from the true faith and pierced [himself or herself] with many sorrows."

The decision to declare what is enough has to be made outside the moment. Waiting until our eyes see the food or our hunger pangs speak up is too late to wisely decide on what's enough. If old habits of letting desires decide are deeply ingrained, the wise decision may require us to stay away from the places where we know our desires will get the opportunity to take charge the wrong way. The power to abstain often preserves contentment!

DISCUSSION QUESTIONS ABOUT SCRIPTURE

❖ Why is contentment a wiser option than relief?

_____

_____

_____

_____

_____

_____

❖ What does "enough" mean to you?

_____

_____

_____

_____

_____

❖ What's the difference between "discovery" and "decision" when it comes to deciding on "enough"?

_____

_____

_____

_____

_____

_____

❖ Why does God urge us to be content?

_____

_____

_____

_____

_____

❖ What's the connection between "godliness" and "contentment"?

_____

_____

_____

_____

_____

_____

_____

❖ When is this a struggle for you?

_____

_____

_____

_____

_____

_____

_____

CASE STUDY

SAEKO

"Look! The dress is still there." Saeko clutched Jaleesa's arm, then pulled her by the store window. "I love that dress. I wish I could wear that dress for the high school reunion next month. That looks like the size I used to wear."

"Are we walking today or window shopping?" Jaleesa asked.

"I haven't worn it since Aiko was born," Saeko said wistfully. "All the latest styles look better in a smaller size." She set off walking at a pace to which Jaleesa almost had to run to catch up. "I'd hate for everyone at the reunion to look at me and think 'She's gained weight!'"

Jaleesa murmured reassurances, but Saeko wasn't listening. "I want to go back to the way I was. Maybe I should try that new diet shake," Saeko said. "It's supposed to take the pounds off quickly. That's what the infomercial said."

"I heard you gain it right back."

"Who cares, as long as I can lose weight quickly!"

YOUR TURN

❖ Why is Saeko so taken by the dress in the store window?

_____

_____

_____

_____

❖ Why does Saeko want to go back to the way she was in high school?

_____

_____

_____

_____

❖ How does she plan to regain that size, to lose the necessary weight?

_____

_____

_____

_____

❖ Why are Saeko's expectations unrealistic?

_____

_____

_____

_____

_____

AS A GROUP

❖ In what areas do people commonly have unrealistic expectations? Why?

_____

_____

_____

_____

❖ How do these expectations affect our desire for more? In other words, why do we never seem to have enough?

_____

_____

_____

_____

_____

_____

❖ Why should we be content?

_____

_____

_____

_____

_____

_____

❖ How does contentment relate to the need to change, to improve?

_____

_____

_____

_____

_____

CHALLENGE

In reflecting on their many moves during their marriage, one couple explained: "I [the husband] always seem to like where we'll be going next better than where we are. She [the wife] seems to like where we've been better." Obviously, they were struggling with contentment.

Discontentment means not appreciating what we have and always wanting more. It involves comparing ourselves with others or with an ideal. It looks for quick results. And it certainly feeds off unrealistic expectations.

Ask God to help you form realistic goals, to help you decide on what is enough, to give you the strength and motivation to do what you must, and to be content in Him.

DAILY DEVOTIONAL JOURNAL

DAY 1

Scripture: 2 CORINTHIANS 12:8–10

Three different times I begged the Lord to take it away. Each time he said, "My grace is all you need. My power works best in weakness." So now I am glad to boast about my weaknesses, so that the power of Christ can work through me. That's why I take pleasure in my weaknesses, and in the insults, hardships, persecutions, and troubles that I suffer for Christ. For when I am weak, then I am strong.

DEVOTIONAL THOUGHT

When you're in pain, you want a quick solution to the problem. Back hurts? The ibuprofen better work. Emotional pain? The emotional ibuprofen needs to work too. But sometimes God allows pain to remain, as He did in Paul's life. God's purposes are far greater than we could ever dream. "'My thoughts are nothing like your thoughts,' says the LORD. 'And my ways are far beyond anything you could imagine'" (Isaiah 55:8).

Although contentment in weakness is difficult to consider when the pain level grows, it is possible. When pain relief doesn't come, are you, like Paul, willing to surrender your agenda and embrace God's?

Think about the situations where you feel weakest or the prayers that don't seem to have been answered. Are you willing to accept God's words, "My grace is all you need"?

TRUTH I WILL FOCUS ON TODAY

_____

_____

_____

_____

MY PRAYER

_____

_____

_____

_____

DAY 2

Scripture: PHILIPPIANS 4:11–12

Not that I was ever in need, for I have learned to be content with whatever I have. I know how to live on almost nothing or with everything. I have learned the secret of living in every situation, whether it is with a full stomach or empty, with plenty or little.

DEVOTIONAL THOUGHT

Ever play the "if only" game? "If only I had more money, life would be sweet." "If only I could lose those last extra pounds, then I would be content." With the "if only" thoughts crowding our minds, we find ourselves living for the future, rather than in the now.

The apostle Paul knew the secret to satisfaction. It is one word: *contentment*. He was content no matter what circumstance he found himself in. Now most people, if we're honest, will admit that contentment seems like a pipe dream sometimes. But contentment is possible. Just ask the Author of it—the Spirit of God.

TRUTH I WILL FOCUS ON TODAY

_____

_____

_____

_____

MY PRAYER

_____

_____

_____

_____

DAY 3

Scripture: ROMANS 8:23–25

And we believers also groan, even though we have the Holy Spirit within us as a foretaste of future glory, for we long for our bodies to be released from sin and suffering. We, too, wait with eager hope for the day when God will give us our full rights as his adopted children, including the new bodies he has promised us. We were given this hope when we were saved. (If we already have something, we don't need to hope for it. But if we look forward to something we don't yet have, we must wait patiently and confidently.)

DEVOTIONAL THOUGHT

Patience is a fruit of the Spirit for which we seldom ask. Although we need patience, we don't want to have to wait for it! We want it right now! We have the same attitude concerning some of our requests to the Lord. "Lord, I really need you to answer right away." We don't want *the hope* of His answer. We want *the answer*, especially if we're suffering.

Waiting activates the trust mechanism within us. It reminds us of our dependence on God. Do we really trust that God has our best interests at heart? If so, "we must wait patiently and confidently."

For what are you hoping? Ask the Lord to help you wait patiently and confidently until He answers.

TRUTH I WILL FOCUS ON TODAY

_____

_____

_____

_____

MY PRAYER

_____

_____

_____

_____

DAY 4

Scripture: **PHILIPPIANS 1:20**

For I fully expect and hope that I will never be ashamed, but that I will continue to be bold for Christ, as I have been in the past. And I trust that my life will bring honor to Christ, whether I live or die.

DEVOTIONAL THOUGHT

When life takes a hard turn, our beliefs about God are put to the test. A tragedy can shake us to the core. We reel, wondering where God is or why He allowed such pain in our lives.

The apostle Paul's missionary life was difficult to say the least. But he short-circuited the desire to doubt by plugging into a prayer for boldness no matter what the circumstance. *Whether I live or die*—no matter what course life takes. Is that your prayer? Why not make it your prayer today?

TRUTH I WILL FOCUS ON TODAY

_____

_____

_____

_____

MY PRAYER

_____

_____

_____

_____

DAY 5

Scripture: HEBREWS 11:1

Faith is the confidence that what we hope for will actually happen; it gives us assurance about things we cannot see.

DEVOTIONAL THOUGHT

Picture a diver leaping off a board or a high cliff. He or she arcs gracefully before plunging into the water below. Sometimes faith can seem like that—a plunge into what you hope lies below. But faith is what causes you to take the plunge in the first place, instead of remaining on the diving board or the cliff.

You've heard the old saying that "faith is not a feeling." We sometimes wait for a feeling of confident assurance before taking a step of faith. That's like diving and trying to hold onto the board at the same time. You can't do both.

What step of faith are you considering? What are you holding on to: your faith in your faith, or a confident assurance of God's love for you?

TRUTH I WILL FOCUS ON TODAY

_____

_____

_____

_____

MY PRAYER

_____

_____

_____

_____

DAY 6

Scripture: **HEBREWS 10:1**

The old system under the law of Moses was only a shadow, a dim preview of the good things to come, not the good things themselves. The sacrifices under that system were repeated again and again, year after year, but they were never able to provide perfect cleansing for those who came to worship.

DEVOTIONAL THOUGHT

Some ways of compensating only work for a season. We try to "make do" with substitutes until we can get "the real thing." In the Old Testament, sacrifices were only a substitute payment for the price of sin. But they were not the ultimate sacrifice. Only Jesus—the perfect sacrifice—could completely pay the price of sin.

In what ways do you find yourself compensating as you wait for the answer to a prayer? Perhaps you're finding that your compensation meter is running on empty. While you wait, ask God to renew your strength. Remember: "Those who trust in the Lord will find new strength. They will soar high on wings like eagles. They will run and not grow weary. They will walk and not faint" (Isaiah 40:31).

TRUTH I WILL FOCUS ON TODAY

_____

_____

_____

_____

MY PRAYER

_____

_____

_____

_____

DAY 7

Scripture: 1 PETER 4:19

So if you are suffering in a manner that pleases God, keep on doing what is right, and trust your lives to the God who created you, for he will never fail you.

DEVOTIONAL THOUGHT

No one likes open-ended suffering. But some cycles of suffering can seem endless, and we don't feel like the Energizer Bunny, able to keep going and going. And that's the crux of the matter. We don't *feel* like continuing. That's why the apostle Peter urged his readers to persevere through suffering. How can we persevere? "Trust your lives to the God who created you." *Trust* is the key.

He is your lifeline when the world seems to spin out of control. Are you holding on to Him? "He will never fail you." Do you believe that?

TRUTH I WILL FOCUS ON TODAY

_____

_____

_____

_____

MY PRAYER

_____

_____

_____

_____

WEEKLY PROGRESS AND GOALS

❖ Current weight: _____

❖ Pounds lost this week: _____

NEW INSIGHTS

❖ About myself:

_____

_____

❖ From Scripture:

_____

_____

❖ About weight loss:

_____

_____

PLAN FOR NEXT WEEK

❖ Personal issue to focus on:

_____

_____

❖ Biblical truth to live out:

_____

_____

❖ Food to eliminate or restrict for the week:

_____

_____

❖ Exercise goals:

_____

_____

INTRODUCTION

You've worked hard, pushing yourself to complete twelve-hour workdays. You haven't spent quality time with your family or friends in weeks, but you know that it all will be worth it soon—tomorrow you should learn that you're getting the promotion. As you finish answering your last e-mail, you grab your bag, turn off the lights, and, with confidence, head home.

Arriving at the office the next morning, you anxiously check your messages. Your stomach churns as you wait to meet with your boss. Around noon he calls you in. There, sitting in a chair, is the man who has just stolen your promotion. You've never seen him before—he's just some guy who dropped off his resumé a few weeks ago. Excusing yourself, you rush to the restroom and try to regain your composure.

It's unfair, you think. *I've done everything right, yet they pick someone they don't even know!* Other similar thoughts rush through your mind, and you realize that you've come to a fork in the road. You can choose to let the resentment build and, then, respond in anger, or you can trust in God's plan and allow Him to strengthen you through this situation. The easier response is anger, but the better response is mercy.

How do you respond when life seems unfair?

VIDEO 9

Notes from video:

_____

_____

_____

_____

_____

_____

_____

_____

_____

_____

THE MOST DANGEROUS POSSESSION YOU CAN CARRY THROUGHOUT YOUR LIFE IS JUSTIFIABLE RESENTMENT.

We would be shocked to learn that a friend or neighbor regularly carried a loaded gun, concealed in a briefcase, purse, or jacket. The idea of being so close to such a dangerous weapon would be unnerving. "How could someone do such a thing," we might say, "and put us all at risk?"

Yet dangerous possessions can come in different, subtler forms. Sometimes, when we're wronged (or think we are), we add bitterness and resentment to the emotional backpack. If those feelings are left alone or are nurtured, they can build until they suddenly explode, harming us and everyone nearby.

We may be unfairly singled out for criticism or passed over for a promotion. We may live in the shadow of a favored sibling. We may struggle with less-than-positive news from a doctor. We may just be tired of the continual stream of negative news emanating from the media. Whatever the cause and even if we have "every right to be angry" having been unfairly treated, this resentment is dangerous and must be defused.

SCRIPTURE

GENESIS 4:1–12

Now Adam had sexual relations with his wife, Eve, and she became pregnant. When she gave birth to Cain, she said, "With the LORD's help, I have produced a man!" Later she gave birth to his brother and named him Abel.

When they grew up, Abel became a shepherd, while Cain cultivated the ground. When it was time for the harvest, Cain presented some of his crops as a gift to the LORD. Abel also brought a gift—the best of the firstborn lambs from his flock. The LORD accepted Abel and his gift, but he did not accept Cain and his gift. This made Cain very angry, and he looked dejected.

"Why are you so angry?" the LORD asked Cain. "Why do you look so dejected? You will be accepted if you do what is right. But if you refuse to do what is right, then watch out! Sin is crouching at the door, eager to control you. But you must subdue it and be its master."

One day Cain suggested to his brother, "Let's go out into the fields." And while they were in the field, Cain attacked his brother, Abel, and killed him.

> Afterward the LORD asked Cain, "Where is your brother? Where is Abel?"
>
> "I don't know," Cain responded. "Am I my brother's guardian?"
>
> But the LORD said, "What have you done? Listen! Your brother's blood cries out to me from the ground! Now you are cursed and banished from the ground, which has swallowed your brother's blood. No longer will the ground yield good crops for you, no matter how hard you work! From now on you will be a homeless wanderer on the earth."

The world is a sick and dying place. It may still feature beautiful vistas, heroic moments, and noteworthy achievements, but it is a terminal planet. We will not be able to live in this world and avoid being touched and hurt by the evil that infects our environment. Ecological and natural disasters can't match the relentless harm created by relational chaos in the world. Creation has been unraveling since the beginning, and God will determine when the time has come to bring down the curtain on the universe.

Part of understanding our present condition involves looking back at the origins of the human race and our impact on creation. The original pollution of the earth was sin. Adam and Eve rejected God's direction and brought a willful infection into all the good that God created. That infection (sin) passed into their children, Cain and Abel. In this session's Scripture passage, we see the terrible effects that sin brought about in the human race.

The first two children grew up with an awareness of God but with different attitudes about what God required. Both understood the idea of an honoring sacrifice, but Abel took his sacrificing seriously while Cain took the casual approach. Abel chose the best of his flock; Cain grabbed what was at hand. God accepted Abel's sacrifice and told Cain to try again. Instead, Cain got resentful. It was more than the issue of the sacrifice. God had accepted Abel before accepting his big brother.

God warned Cain that he was walking on dangerous ground. God told him to do "what is right." God didn't chide Cain for his anger, but warned that his resentment was an invitation to sin. Instead of doing what was right, Cain chose to even the score. His resentment became a need that could only be satisfied by eliminating the cause—Abel. So Cain betrayed and killed his own little brother.

What started out as a feeling of unfairness grew into full-blown destructive behavior. Cain illustrated the warning contained in LIFL Concept Nine carried out to its logical and deadly conclusion. In a twisted way, Cain justified his resentment and anger by reasoning that nothing would have happened if Abel hadn't been around to present a more acceptable sacrifice! He clearly didn't grasp the significance of self-made traps (Concept One) and the blindness of lying to oneself (Concept Two).

Cain understood that life included a debt of gratitude to God. Like his brother, he presented a sacrifice, at least dutifully. But his external participation in an expression of worship couldn't hide from God his internal bad attitude. And his reaction to disappointment revealed his inner lack of integrity. Cain had a clear opportunity to make the hard good choice, but he made the sinful choice that destroyed his brother's life, harmed his family, and made his own life chaotic.

Given the degree of danger, one might expect that LIFL Concept Nine would occur earlier in the list. But the kind of lingering and destructive resentment that is addressed by this concept doesn't raise its ugly head until we've come a long way in the other concepts. Perhaps we're applying these concepts and are not making much progress. Or maybe putting into action what we're learning has been a real struggle. Those kinds of setbacks can gradually provoke anger. They can make us resentful over the unfairness of life's unfairnesses. Why doesn't it get easier to do what is right?

Disappointments can make us give up or make us realize that we're in a real life-and-death struggle. LIFL is serious business. And if we give up when things don't go the way we expect, that shows we didn't realize the seriousness of the challenge we were facing. As God told Cain, behind the door of anger and resentment, sin is "crouching … eager to control you" (Genesis 4:7). But God didn't stop with a warning. He added guidance: "But you must subdue it and be its master" (Genesis 4:7). The exact opposite happened. The fact that Cain invited his brother "out into the fields" shows that Abel's murder was premeditated. Cain's plan was fueled by resentment, which Abel may not have even recognized until it was too late.

Concept Nine brings us face-to-face with "justifiable resentment" as a life-long, constant, and dangerous companion. Even when we think we're completely convinced of Concept One and have taken responsibility for the "prisons and chains that trap us and keep us from a life of freedom," we haven't left behind the possibility of more wrong choices. We can accept responsibility one moment and then hand it off to someone else the next. Or we can publicly claim our role while secretly maintaining the conviction that our problems are really someone else's fault. This is because the very capacity we have for taking responsibility can be misused to dodge responsibility. Blaming others (even God) is always a way to deflect responsibility away from ourselves. This tendency showed up in the human race even before Cain. When Adam and Eve were confronted with their sin, they immediately started to play the blame game. Cain was an expert at this game. Not only did he refuse to accept responsibility for his lack of attentive worship, but he also responded to God's question about his brother's whereabouts with, "That's someone else's business, not mine." Sin was in full control.

We live with the same choices that faced Cain. And God wants to help us make the right ones. The ongoing danger of resentment and other challenges is why LIFL (Lose It For Life) isn't LIFAW (Lose It For A While). All of these concepts are applicable daily. We're in this for a lifetime.

DISCUSSION QUESTIONS ABOUT SCRIPTURE

❖ Why do you think Cain was so resentful of Abel?

_____

_____

_____

_____

_____

_____

❖ How do you think that resentment progressed?

_____

_____

_____

_____

_____

_____

❖ What did God mean by His statement to Cain, "Sin is crouching at the door, eager to control you"?

_____

_____

_____

_____

_____

❖ What do you think Cain could have done to "subdue it and be its master"?

_____

_____

_____

_____

_____

❖ In what situations might we be tempted to think our resentment is justified?

_____

_____

_____

_____

_____

❖ How do we face the same choices as Cain?

_____

_____

_____

_____

CASE STUDY

DON

Yep. The old spare tire was still there. A quick look in the mirror showed that. When Don was twenty-five, he could exercise less and still lose weight quickly. But now at forty, an increased amount of exercise seemed to have even *less* results. Plus the new medication he was on made weight loss even harder.

Now his doctor was actually telling him to run *less*. "Ease up a bit. You're putting too much pressure on those knees," he'd said. "You've got that problem with cartilage." Don gave an annoyed sigh. It's not like the doctor didn't still harp on him to lose weight. How was he *ever* to lose weight? He was beginning to feel as if the deck was stacked against him.

When his wife later asked him about his visit to the doctor, he snapped at her and yelled at the kids.

YOUR TURN

❖ What is Don's problem?

_____

_____

_____

_____

❖ Why was he annoyed with the doctor?

_____

_____

_____

_____

_____

_____

❖ How did that annoyance build into resentment?

_____

_____

_____

_____

_____

_____

❖ What caused Don to show anger to his wife and children?

_____

_____

_____

_____

_____

_____

AS A GROUP

❖ What are some common causes for "justifiable resentment"?

_____

_____

_____

_____

_____

❖ What are some typical reasons for resentment for people in LIFL groups?

_____

_____

_____

_____

_____

_____

❖ What might occur if we don't "subdue [resentment] and be its master"?

_____

_____

_____

_____

_____

_____

❖ What can we do to rid ourselves of this possession?

_____

_____

_____

_____

_____

CHALLENGE

What irks you about your situation in life? What circumstances, conversations, or conundrums cause you to feel resentful? Left alone, that resentment can build and become a dangerous weapon, threatening to discharge at any moment and hurt you and others.

Recognize those resentments—name them—and ask God to take them away. Be sure to apologize to anyone who has been on the receiving end of your unexpected explosions.

DAILY DEVOTIONAL JOURNAL

DAY 1

Scripture: EPHESIANS 4:31

Get rid of all bitterness, rage, anger, harsh words, and slander, as well as all types of evil behavior.

DEVOTIONAL THOUGHT

When we're frustrated or tired, our tempers fray. We feel pushed to the edge—ready to say or do something we'll regret. These words of the apostle Paul are a preventative measure—a railing to keep you from going over the edge of anger and into the chasm of deep regret.

Take a look at that phrase. What in that list do you need to get rid of? Prayerfully allow God to sift through the list of your life, and get ready to take out the trash.

TRUTH I WILL FOCUS ON TODAY

_____

_____

_____

_____

MY PRAYER

_____

_____

_____

_____

DAY 2

Scripture: **JOB 36:13**

For the godless are full of resentment. Even when he punishes them, they refuse to cry out to him for help.

DEVOTIONAL THOUGHT

Resentment is the breeding ground for all kinds of trouble. Seasoned with anger, it simmers on the petri dish of our souls until bitterness hatches. In Job 36, a well-meaning Elihu tried to warn Job of the dangers of resentment and a refusal to yield to God's discipline.

If you find resentment simmering, turn down the flame by calling out to God for help. Even if you're angry with Him, are you willing to still talk the matter over with Him?

TRUTH I WILL FOCUS ON TODAY

_____

_____

_____

_____

MY PRAYER

_____

_____

_____

_____

DAY 3

Scripture: PROVERBS 27:3

A stone is heavy and sand is weighty, but the resentment caused by a fool is even heavier.

DEVOTIONAL THOUGHT

If you've ever hoisted a sandbag, you know how heavy sand in mass quantity can be. Isn't it amazing how tiny grains of sand that you might pick up at a beach and sift through your fingers can weigh you down? Resentment is like that. It may seem tiny at first, until we dwell on it. Then it becomes as weighty as the proverbial stone.

This proverb reminds us that running around with resentment is as foolish as trying to run with a large stone strapped to one's back. Resentment is a defense mechanism that sometimes kicks in when we feel helpless. When life seems unfair, we can fall victim to resentment if we're not careful.

Feeling a weight of resentment? The Cross of Christ is nearby. Why not drop it there?

TRUTH I WILL FOCUS ON TODAY

_____

_____

_____

_____

MY PRAYER

_____

_____

_____

_____

DAY 4

Scripture: **LUKE 10:29**

The man wanted to justify his actions, so he asked Jesus, "And who is my neighbor?"

DEVOTIONAL THOUGHT

This man was an expert in religious law—a man of great learning who desired to match wits with Jesus. "Let's see how you answer this," his question couched in resentment seems to imply. Instead, the man found himself outwitted and disarmed by a parable about love.

We may have that "let's see how you answer this" approach to God as well. Staying behind a wall of frustration or resentment is tempting, especially when we're fighting a losing battle (literally and figuratively). We might want to blame God or have our efforts applauded, instead of being told that we're not doing enough or that we're following the wrong agenda. Sometimes God wants us to go beyond the limits we've established for our lives. This may mean going beyond our comfort zone to accomplish a goal we've set.

Tempted to justify your actions? Are you willing to submit them to the Lord and accept His evaluation?

TRUTH I WILL FOCUS ON TODAY

_____

_____

_____

_____

MY PRAYER

_____

_____

_____

_____

DAY 5

Scripture: ISAIAH 58:8

Then your salvation will come like the dawn, and your wounds will quickly heal. Your godliness will lead you forward, and the glory of the LORD will protect you from behind.

DEVOTIONAL THOUGHT

Ever come to resent a word of advice? Perhaps the doctor has warned you to eat less carbs or exercise more. If you follow the doctor's advice, you can expect a good result. But if the efforts involve hard work with few discernible results right away, you might resent the advice.

Throughout the Old Testament, God added cause-and-effect clauses to His commands. "If you do this, expect this result." He stated in Isaiah that if His people lived out their faith by helping the oppressed and hungry, then salvation and healing would come. His rules were not meant to be onerous but to serve as protection, like the rear guard of an army.

What actions do you need to take to affect change in your life? Consider the fact that the Lord acts as your rear guard, shielding you from the harm of poor choices.

TRUTH I WILL FOCUS ON TODAY

_____

_____

_____

_____

MY PRAYER

_____

_____

_____

_____

DAY 6

Scripture: **EPHESIANS 4:26**

And "don't sin by letting anger gain control over you." Don't let the sun go down while you are still angry.

DEVOTIONAL THOUGHT

In this passage, Paul gives a variation on Psalm 4:4: "Don't sin by letting anger control you. Think about it overnight and remain silent." This helps us to dial down anger and prevent it from controlling us.

Resentment is like the constant drip of a faucet. Our annoyance increases the more we dwell on it. It's best to get a handle on it, Paul admonishes, before the end of the day. What do you need to talk over with someone before another day passes?

TRUTH I WILL FOCUS ON TODAY

_____

_____

_____

_____

MY PRAYER

_____

_____

_____

_____

DAY 7

Scripture: JAMES 1:19–20

Understand this, my dear brothers and sisters: You must all be quick to listen, slow to speak, and slow to get angry. Human anger does not produce the righteousness God desires.

DEVOTIONAL THOUGHT

Often in life our experience is the opposite of James's advice. We're quicker to get angry than we are to listen, especially if resentment fuels our remarks or beliefs. God, however, is slow to get angry (see Exodus 34:5). His carefully measured responses are a testament of control and a model to follow.

Anger is as dangerous as a raging forest fire. Once started, it is difficult to put out. With whom are you angry? How can you begin to make things right?

TRUTH I WILL FOCUS ON TODAY

_____

_____

_____

_____

MY PRAYER

_____

_____

_____

_____

WEEKLY PROGRESS AND GOALS

❖ Current weight: _____

❖ Pounds lost this week: _____

NEW INSIGHTS

❖ About myself:

_____

_____

❖ From Scripture:

_____

_____

❖ About weight loss:

_____

_____

PLAN FOR NEXT WEEK

❖ Personal issue to focus on:

_____

_____

❖ Biblical truth to live out:

_____

_____

❖ Food to eliminate or restrict for the week:

_____

_____

❖ Exercise goals:

_____

_____

INTRODUCTION

A parasite lives off its "host," slowly sapping it of life and energy. The process is slow and almost undetectable. It may go unnoticed for a long while, but eventually the damaging, often deadly, effects to the host are obvious.

Thankfully, most of us are not carrying around real parasites. However, we may still experience the effects of being "eaten away" on the inside. That's how some of our hidden emotions can affect us. Bitterness and shame, for example, can eat away at us—body and soul. At first this may not be obvious. But as we feed these feelings (and, many times, our stomachs as well), the problem becomes apparent, often through weight gain and other issues. Holding on to resentment causes it to grow, and consequently, causes more harm emotionally.

But we can stop this process. When we forgive others and accept God's forgiveness, God begins to heal us and reverse the damage we've inflicted on ourselves.

VIDEO 10

Notes from video:

_____

_____

_____

_____

_____

_____

_____

_____

_____

_____

_____

_____

_____

_____

_____

LIFL CONCEPT 10

RATHER THAN FEED RESENTMENT OR ALLOW BITTERNESS TO EAT AT US, OR US EAT AT IT, WE MUST WORK TO FORGIVE AND RELEASE THOSE WHO HAVE HURT US SO THAT WE MAY LIVE FREE.

The last session focused on the danger of carrying justifiable resentment and the fact that it may explode at any moment, harming us and those closest to us. And we discussed asking God for guidance and power to help us let go of those feelings, justified or not.

In this session, we see another internal enemy that threatens to harm us and keep us from reaching our goals. Instead of an explosion, however, this enemy is a silent killer, consuming us from the inside.

Regardless of why we have been wronged or the severity of the offense, bitterness and unforgiveness can eat us alive and prevent us from achieving our goals. The only way to stop this parasitic killer is by forgiving ourselves and others. Only then will we be able to live in freedom.

SCRIPTURE

EPHESIANS 4:20–32

But that isn't what you learned about Christ. Since you have heard about Jesus and have learned the truth that comes from him, throw off your old sinful nature and your former way of life, which is corrupted by lust and deception. Instead, let the Spirit renew your thoughts and attitudes. Put on your new nature, created to be like God—truly righteous and holy.

So stop telling lies. Let us tell our neighbors the truth, for we are all parts of the same body. And "don't sin by letting anger control you." Don't let the sun go down while you are still angry, for anger gives a foothold to the devil.

If you are a thief, quit stealing. Instead, use your hands for good hard work, and then give generously to others in need. Don't use foul language. Let everything you say be good and helpful, so that your words will be an encouragement to those who hear them.

And do not bring sorrow to God's Holy Spirit by the way you live. Remember, he has identified you as his own, guaranteeing that you will be saved on the day of redemption.

> **Get rid of all bitterness, rage, anger, harsh words, and slander, as well as all types of evil behavior. Instead, be kind to each other, tenderhearted, forgiving one another, just as God through Christ has forgiven you.**

If this passage seems familiar, you're right! We looked at it in some detail when we discussed Concept Six. We focused in that session on the development of a "training" mindset in exchange for our usual "trying" mindset. This passage teaches a pattern we can use in dealing with habits and behaviors that we know are keeping us from experiencing freedom. The three actions in this training plan can be summarized as: *throw off* (verse 22), *be renewed* (verse 23), and *put on* (verse 24).

We learned that these verses also include five case studies to help us see the pattern in operation. The case studies highlight problems with lying, anger, stealing, foul language, and abusive behaviors. These are relational issues involving the way we treat other people or the Holy Spirit. Most of us are in training in one or more of these areas. Like repeated exercises or laps around the course, we are deliberately and prayerfully "putting off" these things, breathing in a renewed sense of God's Spirit at work in us, and "putting on" the opposite behaviors from the ones we're rejecting. We're replacing anger with peacemaking, eliminating stealing and putting on hard work and generosity, replacing harsh words with helpful ones, and rejecting uncaring and abusive treatment of others with an attitude of forgiveness.

This last mark of progress, the growing capacity for forgiveness, serves not only as the "putting on" part of the last case study but also as a summary of our ultimate purpose in relationships.

Knowing Jesus Christ raises the bar in relationships. The "Golden Rule" that Jesus taught us turns into the "Platinum Rule" in Ephesians 4:32. Jesus said that the basic standard of relationships with others ought to be, "Do to others whatever you would like them to do to you. This is the essence of all that is taught in the law and the prophets" (Matthew 7:12). All that Jesus accomplished for us means that we must go beyond the base standard.

Paul wrote, "Be kind to each other, tenderhearted, forgiving one another, just as God through Christ has forgiven you." Thus, expanding on Jesus' words, the Platinum Rule tells us, "Do for others what *Jesus has done* for you." This is particularly true when we have applied the Golden Rule to a relationship only to have that person treat us poorly in return. Without Christ's example, violations of the Golden Rule often result in the "Eye for an Eye Rule"—as in, "I was kind to you. You were mean to me. So now you're going to get it!" But Christ practiced the Golden Rule perfectly and was still rejected. In a vivid moment of that rejection, as Jesus was nailed to the cross and raised up between earth and sky, He applied the Platinum Rule and said, "Father, forgive them for they don't know what they are doing" (Luke 23:34).

Given the kind of world we live in, it's safe to say that the health of any relationship can be measured by the degree of forgiveness in that relationship. Offenses are unavoidable;

forgiveness is a choice. Misunderstandings, sins, and hurts are daily occurrences, so we need to stock up on forgiveness in our relationships.

One helpful picture is to identify forgiveness as the "white blood cells" in our relationships. The red blood cells are love. White bloods cells are adaptable, sacrificial cells that immediately surround and isolate infections and foreign bodies in our system. When harm invades the relationship in any form, forgiveness cells are the first responders, rushing to the scene.

Our relationship with Christ grows as we come to appreciate more and more just how much He has forgiven us. When we lose sight of that for a moment, we tend to become less forgiving of others and ourselves. At the human level, forgiveness is often reduced to an even exchange: "I'll forgive you and hope you'll forgive me. But I may not forgive you until I get a sign that you will forgive me." But Christ's example goes far beyond that. It initiates forgiveness without demanding an exchange. In our relationship with Him *no exchange* occurs. We can't hold anything over Him upon which to demand His forgiveness. We are only offenders—that's all—and we come to Christ each day with the promise that He has already forgiven. We simply accept that forgiveness.

Christ's unique form of one-sided forgiveness puts all of our challenges to forgive in a special light, the light of the Platinum Rule. If we have accepted Christ's forgiveness, then the need to forgive ourselves and others takes on different authority. We no longer have any excuse for not forgiving someone and using that to justify our actions. We simply need to obey Jesus' words and forgive ourselves and others as He has forgiven us.

Think for a moment of the variety of destructive behaviors we engage in that are actually based on unforgiveness. Our longing for forgiveness sometimes get translated into all kinds of other hungers. But no food, pleasure, or person can meet and satisfy the deep hunger we have for forgiveness from God. Christ's forgiveness can supply a lifetime of wonder in reflection and power in action. We will never exhaust Christ's forgiveness by passing it on to others—even to ourselves.

One of the most moving scenes in the New Testament involves a woman who approached Jesus during a meal and washed His feet with her tears. The religiously pious people were appalled that Jesus would let a sinful woman even touch Him. But He saw her actions as pure love. Jesus said, "I tell you, her sins—and they are many—have been forgiven, so she has shown me much love. But a person who is forgiven little shows only little love" (Luke 7:47). The challenging point is that our actions mirror our understanding of forgiveness. When we can't or won't forgive ourselves and others, we simply show that we don't understand the forgiveness God has offered us. But the more we appreciate and let ourselves be overwhelmed with God's grace and forgiveness toward us, the more others will benefit from the forgiveness that will flow from us.

DISCUSSION QUESTIONS ABOUT SCRIPTURE

❖ What is your understanding of the Golden Rule?

_____

_____

_____

_____

_____

❖ How does it differ from the "Platinum Rule"?

_____

_____

_____

_____

_____

❖ Why does Jesus forgive us when we have nothing to offer Him in exchange?

_____

_____

_____

_____

_____

❖ How does that make us feel? How should we respond?

_____

_____

_____

_____

❖ What can we do to "put on" forgiveness?

_____

_____

_____

_____

❖ What makes forgiving others so difficult?

_____

_____

_____

_____

_____

❖ Why is it so difficult to forgive ourselves?

_____

_____

_____

_____

❖ In what ways does unforgiveness harm us? How does forgiveness help us?

_____

_____

_____

_____

CASE STUDY

DIEDRE

Diedre loved her mother, she reminded herself. But her mother's remarks about her weight continued to rankle.

"Honey, your sister is wondering what size she should order for your maid of honor dress," her mother said on the phone one day. "I told her your weight goes up and down so much, it's hard for me to say."

"I'll call her later," Diedre said through gritted teeth.

"Why don't you try the new diet they talked about on the news yesterday? It's supposed to get better results than you've gotten lately."

"I'm doing just fine, Mother!"

"Well, I'm only trying to help. You're so touchy these days. No one can talk to you."

"Mom! Stay out of this, okay?" Diedre yelled, before hanging up the phone. _She always does this to me,_ she fumed.

YOUR TURN

❖ Why was Diedre upset with her mother?

_____

_____

_____

_____

❖ What triggered her outburst on the phone?

_____

_____

_____

_____

❖ What was the root cause of Diedre's anger?

_____

_____

_____

_____

❖ What might be the role of forgiveness in this situation?

_____

_____

_____

_____

AS A GROUP

❖ For what personal offenses might we refuse to forgive someone?

_____

_____

_____

❖ What people might be most difficult to forgive?

_____

_____

_____

❖ Why can bitterness and withholding forgiveness lead to emotional eating? In what other ways might this hurt us?

_____

_____

_____

_____

❖ What will it take to forgive someone who has hurt or wronged you deeply?

_____

_____

_____

_____

CHALLENGE

Certainly you have been hurt—everyone has. Whether the cause of the wound was as minor as a verbal insult or as major as a betrayal, we can feel justified in holding onto feeling bitter toward the one who has wounded us. And often the offender is a person close to us: spouse, parent, sibling, friend, church member, co-worker, or neighbor. In most cases we assume that this person _meant_ to hurt us through their fault-finding, nagging, promise-breaking, reputation-damaging, insulting, or similar actions. Feeling bitter and angry and refusing to forgive are natural responses to those kinds of transgressions. But they destroy relationships and boomerang, inflicting hurt on those who hold such attitudes.

The only person in history with the absolute right to be bitter was Jesus. Just think about it. He never sinned. He loved people and spoke the truth. Yet He was falsely accused, abandoned by friends, convicted in an illegal trial, and condemned to death. And approaching death, in excruciating pain, one of His last statements was forgiveness for the people who put Him there, and by extension, for all of us whose sins put Him on that cross. If Jesus could forgive us, shouldn't we be able to forgive others? No one deserves God's forgiveness—not even you—yet we can have it free through Christ because He paid the price for our sin with His life.

Forgive yourself. Forgive those who have wronged and hurt you. Release them. Exterminate the parasite of bitterness that lives within.

DAILY DEVOTIONAL JOURNAL

DAY 1

Scripture: MATTHEW 6:14–15

If you forgive those who sin against you, your heavenly Father will forgive you.
But if you refuse to forgive others, your Father will not forgive your sins.

DEVOTIONAL THOUGHT

Some wrongs are a constant irritation. They rub at us and rub at us. If we allow resentment in, a hard pellet of bitterness results. But if we mix in forgiveness, a pearl results. Jesus' words here are a stern warning to any who would harbor unforgiveness or resentment. We cannot expect forgiveness if we refuse to forgive.

Who needs the release of your forgiveness? Perhaps this is someone who has doubted your ability to lose weight or who embarrasses you about it. Ask God to help you forgive.

TRUTH I WILL FOCUS ON TODAY

_____

_____

_____

_____

MY PRAYER

_____

_____

_____

_____

DAY 2

Scripture: MATTHEW 18:21–22

Then Peter came to him and asked, "Lord, how often should I forgive someone who sins against me? Seven times?" "No, not seven times," Jesus replied, "seventy times seven!"

DEVOTIONAL THOUGHT

Rabbinic teaching allowed a person to forgive another person up to three times for the same offense. So Peter, who hoped to be generous, must have been flabbergasted when Jesus added an exponent to the number. "How about an unlimited amount of times?" Jesus' words imply. In other words, don't stop forgiving.

Ever find yourself stuck on a number for forgiveness? Consider the fact that God offers forgiveness every time we need it. He also gives us grace to forgive, even when we find forgiving most difficult. Have you asked Him for that grace lately?

TRUTH I WILL FOCUS ON TODAY

_____

_____

_____

_____

MY PRAYER

_____

_____

_____

_____

DAY 3

Scripture: MARK 11:24–25

I tell you, you can pray for anything, and if you believe that you've received it, it will be yours. But when you are praying, first forgive anyone you are holding a grudge against, so that your Father in heaven will forgive your sins, too.

DEVOTIONAL THOUGHT

God's love is unconditional. His forgiveness is offered freely. *But* we are forgiven as freely as we offer forgiveness. We can't hold on to unforgiveness and reach for God's forgiveness at the same time.

Jesus' words are also a blueprint for effective prayer. Our prayers are hindered when we hold on to a grudge. It's like sheltering a raging flame in our cupped hands. Sooner or later, it will burn us.

If you have been praying for something and wondering why you haven't heard an answer, check the forgiveness factor. Is there someone you've put off forgiving? Are you willing to talk to God about it?

TRUTH I WILL FOCUS ON TODAY

_____

_____

_____

MY PRAYER

_____

_____

_____

_____

DAY 4

Scripture: LUKE 6:37

Do not judge others, and you will not be judged. Do not condemn others, or it will all come back against you. Forgive others, and you will be forgiven.

DEVOTIONAL THOUGHT

Which rises quickest to your lips: a compliment or a criticism? Most of us, if we're honest, would say the latter. Jesus, who was constantly surrounded by the critical Pharisees, warned His disciples against such judgmental behavior. He instead explained the reciprocal nature of forgiveness.

Sometimes we're most critical or unforgiving of ourselves. Are you holding a grudge against yourself for not reaching a goal as fast as you would have liked? Or perhaps you're stuck in the mire of "if only." *If only I hadn't eaten that. . . . If only I weren't such a procrastinator.* Can you relate to the voice of criticism? If so, why not ask the Holy Spirit to help you forgive even your worst critic: you.

TRUTH I WILL FOCUS ON TODAY

_____

_____

_____

_____

MY PRAYER

_____

_____

_____

_____

DAY 5

Scripture: 2 CORINTHIANS 2:7–8

Now, however, it is time to forgive and comfort him. Otherwise he may be overcome by discouragement. So I urge you now to reaffirm your love for him.

DEVOTIONAL THOUGHT

Paul admonished the Corinthian believers to forgive a fellow believer whose sin was made public. Now was the time for encouragement instead of blame. *Easier said than done,* we think, when we are contemplating wrongs done to us for which we're still in recovery.

As with anything in our Christian walk, God promises to empower us to do what He calls us to do. Do you believe He will do that for you? Ask God for renewed love and grace to extend forgiveness and even affirmation to someone in your life.

TRUTH I WILL FOCUS ON TODAY

_____
_____
_____
_____

MY PRAYER

_____
_____
_____
_____

DAY 6

Scripture: COLOSSIANS 3:13

Make allowance for each other's faults, and forgive anyone who offends you. Remember, the Lord forgave you, so you must forgive others.

DEVOTIONAL THOUGHT

We know our faults pretty well and would like others (including God) to cut us some slack concerning them. But what about the faults of others? In his letter Paul urged believers in and around the trading city of Colosse to practice forbearance and forgiveness. Knowing that others are as imperfect as we are makes us less quick to judge and faster on the forgiveness draw.

Are forbearance and an increased desire to forgive among the goals you've set for making changes in your life? Why not make those your goals today?

TRUTH I WILL FOCUS ON TODAY

_____

_____

_____

_____

MY PRAYER

_____

_____

_____

_____

DAY 7

Scripture: HEBREWS 8:12

I will forgive their wickedness, and I will never again remember their sins.

DEVOTIONAL THOUGHT

"I can forgive, but I can't forget." Ever say those words? Some offenses seem too deep for us to ever forget. But God says that He not only forgives, He forgets. Here the writer of Hebrews quotes the Lord's words spoken through the prophet Jeremiah (see Jeremiah 31:34). Israel's list of offenses went back centuries. But God willingly wiped the slate clean.

Forgetting does not mean completely erasing our memory of what happened. It means we no longer hold the person accountable for the wrong. Is there someone who still has a list of charges on the blackboard of your life? Are you willing to wipe the slate clean?

TRUTH I WILL FOCUS ON TODAY

_____

_____

_____

_____

MY PRAYER

_____

_____

_____

_____

WEEKLY PROGRESS AND GOALS

❖ Current weight: _____

❖ Pounds lost this week: _____

NEW INSIGHTS

❖ About myself:

_____

_____

❖ From Scripture:

_____

_____

❖ About weight loss:

_____

_____

PLAN FOR NEXT WEEK

❖ Personal issue to focus on:

_____

_____

❖ Biblical truth to live out:

_____

_____

❖ Food to eliminate or restrict for the week:

_____

_____

❖ Exercise goals:

_____

_____

INTRODUCTION

What's easier: singing in the shower or singing a solo at Carnegie Hall? If you've never had any vocal training or have never even sung in front of people before, just thinking about the prospect of performing for a huge audience probably would make your palms sweat. You know that soloing for your first time in that setting could cause emotional scarring and keep you from doing anything like that ever again.

So let's say that instead of jumping into scheduling a concert (or rejecting it outright), you decide to develop your vocal and performance skills and prepare. You begin by taking voice lessons. After a few months of lessons and with the encouragement of your teacher, you gather your courage and sing in a recital. Slowly over the months and years, you build your confidence and work toward bigger audiences. Eventually, these small, incremental changes create in you the desire to be a singer for life—perhaps even with Carnegie Hall in your sights.

The same process works in your healing. The goal, the end result—such as losing lots of weight, forgiving your mother, or interacting in certain social settings—can seem intimidating. But by breaking the long journey into smaller steps, your goal can become attainable and sustainable.

VIDEO 11

Notes from video:

_____

_____

_____

_____

_____

_____

_____

_____

_____

_____

LIFL CONCEPT 11

It is far better to make small changes you can continue for the rest of your life than to make drastic changes you can only maintain for a short time before you turn away and back to your old ways.

Little children often think in terms of *all* or *nothing*—no in between. If Mom says no candy till after dinner, they may just hear the "no" and then respond as though the answer meant "forever." If Dad explains that because of bad weather they can't go to the park, they may think he means they can never go. This tendency appears with timing as well. They want a treat or special event or other desired goal *now*. Waiting isn't an option.

We adults think and act similarly when, feeling pressured to reach a desired goal as soon as possible, we make sudden and drastic changes—all or nothing. That would almost be like competing in a marathon without doing the three-month preparation, singing the National Anthem at Wrigley Field without ever taking a voice lesson, or suiting up for the Patriots' offensive line when you've never played a down of football. Taking this kind of approach to weight loss, we might suddenly begin eating like a sparrow in an effort to drop fifty pounds as quickly as possible.

In each of these scenarios, not only would we find success virtually impossible to attain, but we probably would quit that endeavor (running, singing, playing, or trying to lose weight), never to try again. A much more reasonable and successful approach would be to make small, incremental, and sustainable changes that will move us toward our goal.

SCRIPTURE

MATTHEW 7:24–27

Anyone who listens to my teaching and follows it is wise, like a person who builds a house on solid rock. Though the rain comes in torrents and the floodwaters rise and the winds beat against the house, it won't collapse because it is built on bedrock. But anyone who hears my teaching and ignores it is foolish, like a person who builds a house on sand. When the rains and floods come and the winds beat against that house, it will collapse with a mighty crash.

Jesus knew that when it comes to building a house, as with most areas of life, having knowledge about house-building is not nearly as important as how you actually build it. In the same way, being a certified expert on relationships in not nearly as important as how you actually relate to others. It doesn't matter if you have memorized all the LIFL Concepts if you haven't applied them to your life.

This vivid picture of house-building and natural disasters is a one of Jesus' best-known parables, but people often forget where He gave it. The story appears at the close of what we know as the Sermon on the Mount in Matthew 5–7. In this sermon we find illustrations of many of the LIFL Concepts. Jesus touched on over thirty specific life issues in that sermon. He concluded His speaking by reminding the audience that at that moment they all fit into one category—they had all heard His teaching. But what they would *do* with that teaching would eventually reveal two kinds of people in the audience: the "wise" who would follow Jesus' teaching, and the "foolish" who would ignore it. Everyone would build a life, either on Christ and His words or on a foundation of his or her own choosing.

Jesus also predicted "storms" in the people's lives. In one way or another, they would all experience the torrential rains, floodwaters, and winds of life. The house (life) each one of them built would either stand or fall, depending on the foundation they chose.

This part of Jesus' story may expose a significant misunderstanding on our part. We may have taken up the LIFL challenge because we assumed that the LIFL Concepts would help us avoid many problems in life. But if we still will have to deal with "bad weather," then is the effort worth it? Shouldn't we be looking for a plan that yields a trouble-free, pain-free, struggle-free life?

The truth is that there's not much left to this life if trouble, pain, and struggle are removed. Our experiences with these storms are part and parcel of the weather of a good life. Trouble, pain, and struggle can lead to disaster, but they can also lead to victory, contentment, and meaning. A house that can't stand up to life's storms isn't worth living in.

Those who build their own homes are often advised, "The integrity of a house rests on the integrity of the foundation. If the foundation isn't true (straight and level), everything you build on top of that foundation will be at risk. If you're not sure that you can pour or lay up a plumb foundation, get someone who can." During and after the house is built, that foundation lays beneath, hidden. But the stronger the foundation, the longer a house will stand secure through the seasons.

Jesus claimed that building a life on Him and His teaching will produce a strong life that can outlast any stormy onslaught. Those who ignore Jesus can't rightly blame Him when they are standing in the wreckage of their lives.

The LIFL Concepts are life-building skills based on Christ's teaching. They can be picked up instantly like a tool, but it takes time to build them into a life. Houses aren't built in a day, and neither are our lives. Jesus knew that the proof of His teaching might be felt instantly, but the true effects would only be seen through the passage of time.

Short television programs and the power of time-lapse photography can trick us into thinking that extreme changes can occur rapidly. We assume people can be physically made over and that houses can be magically rebuilt. But in most cases, haste doesn't produce lasting change. And extreme changes that seem to occur painlessly and immediately seldom stand up to the tests of time or the storms of life. The longer a structure is intended to last, the more care is taken in the construction.

The LIFL Concepts are intended for life-long practice. They become part of the daily pattern. Their power and truth is seldom proven by what happens in a single day but by what happens over weeks, months, and years. Those who insist on either instant change or nothing usually end up with nothing. Those who submit to the training of Christ's teaching discover that the storms of life are not to be feared but faced. We know the integrity of the foundation—Christ. He forms an immovable, rock-like solid basis for living.

So read through the Sermon on the Mount and review the LIFL Concepts you've learned to this point. Think about the little, real changes you can begin making. What will you do to live out Christ's words each and every day for the rest of your life? Now that's building a house you can live in!

DISCUSSION QUESTIONS ABOUT SCRIPTURE

❖ What statements or lessons from the Sermon on the Mount mean the most to you right now?

_____

_____

_____

_____

❖ Why do you think Jesus' listeners would appreciate the parable of the builders?

_____

_____

_____

_____

❖ What is the difference between the wise builder and the foolish builder?

_____

_____

_____

_____

❖ What might cause us to build foolishly in our lives?

_____

_____

_____

_____

_____

_____

❖ What does a solid foundation for our lives look like? On what should we be building our lives?

_____

_____

_____

_____

_____

_____

❖ What storms might assault you in the next few years?

_____

_____

_____

_____

_____

_____

❖ What steps can you take now to be able to withstand those storms?

_____

_____

_____

_____

_____

_____

_____

CASE STUDY

JASON

"You what?!" Deborah asked.

"I signed up to run the 10K charity race on Saturday," Jason repeated, slower this time. "What's wrong?" he asked after a pause, noting her disbelieving look.

"You didn't finish the 5K six months ago. The *5K,* Jason," Deborah said with heavy emphasis.

That was old news and twenty pounds ago. Jason felt great now. "So what's your point?" he quipped.

"My point is that you only run a mile or two twice a week now, Jason! You haven't really trained. I'm worried about this sudden change in your routine."

Jason didn't know what his wife was going on about. He was supposed to be trying to lose weight wasn't he? This was the perfect way to do it quickly. If he could run two miles twice a week, he could certainly run a little over six miles. He was in reasonably good shape. Last night's run was great. No problems. Yeah, he could do this. He didn't know why she was so worried.

YOUR TURN

❖ Why did Jason sign up for the 10K race? What did he hope to accomplish?

_____

_____

_____

_____

_____

_____

❖ Why was Deborah so surprised at Jason?

_____

_____

_____

_____

_____

_____

❖ How do you think Jason will do in the race?

_____

_____

_____

_____

_____

_____

❖ What would be a better course of action for Jason?

_____

_____

_____

_____

_____

_____

AS A GROUP

❖ In what areas do people usually want a quick fix?

_____

_____

_____

_____

_____

_____

❖ Why don't we like the idea of taking the time to lay a solid foundation, to take small, incremental steps toward change?

_____

_____

_____

_____

_____

❖ Why is it easier to maintain, over a lifetime, small changes rather than drastic ones?

_____

_____

_____

_____

❖ What small steps might a person take to be able to compete in and finish a 10K race? What small steps might a person take to lose forty pounds?

_____

_____

_____

_____

CHALLENGE

In a previous session, we discussed setting realistic goals, and that's critically important. Equally important, however, is planning on realistic *means* for reaching those goals. Unfortunately, throughout our lives we've been conditioned to expect quick results. We have "instant" foods, drive-thru services, microwave ovens, and access to all sorts of information whenever we want it through the Internet. Our phones, PDAs, and computers keep us in constant contact with friends. So the idea of having to invest time and effort long-term doesn't sound or feel right, and we fall for fad diets and get-in-shape-quick schemes.

But some things can't be hurried: the growth of an oak tree, building a relationship, the formation of a reputation, the crafting of a masterpiece . . . all of these take time.

Developing new habits and changing lifestyles also take time. When we try to meet goals in those areas by jumping too quickly and too far, we may succeed once in a while, but usually we will fall back into our old ways. Instead, we need to build on the rock. We need to move in the right direction steadily, a determined step at a time. Then before we know it, we'll reach that goal! Think of what you can do to build a solid foundation *for life*.

DAILY DEVOTIONAL JOURNAL

DAY 1

Scripture: HABAKKUK 2:2–3

Then the LORD said to me, "Write my answer plainly on tablets, so that a runner can carry the correct message to others. This vision is for a future time. It describes the end, and it will be fulfilled. If it seems slow in coming, wait patiently, for it will surely take place. It will not be delayed."

DEVOTIONAL THOUGHT

God wanted the people of Judah to wait for His answer, rather than run ahead under a mistaken assumption. Yet how many times do we do just that? We want to make major changes in our lives, but we're tempted to run before we can even crawl. Running ahead is especially tempting when an answer to prayer seems a long time in coming.

The apostle Paul has this advice: "If we look forward to something we don't yet have, we must wait patiently and confidently" (Romans 8:25). The apostle Peter also advises, "Supplement your faith . . . with self-control, and self-control with patient endurance, and patient endurance with godliness" (2 Peter 1:5–6). If you're waiting for an answer to prayer, meditate on these words. What do you sense the Lord is saying to you?

TRUTH I WILL FOCUS ON TODAY

_____

_____

_____

_____

MY PRAYER

_____

_____

_____

_____

DAY 2

Scripture: JOB 6:11

But I don't have the strength to endure. I have nothing to live for.

DEVOTIONAL THOUGHT

Job's life was a textbook example of suffering. Here he says, in essence, "I simply don't have the will to continue." Grief or hardship can make us feel like that. We may think we have to manufacture the will to go on, even though we lack a clear-cut goal or direction. Often we wind up spinning our wheels and feeling overwhelmed.

Losing weight can seem just as overwhelming. When we just focus on the problem (the large amount of weight we need to lose), we'll find our energy sapped. When that happens, God advises us to switch our focus. "You will keep in perfect peace all who trust in you, all whose thoughts are fixed on you!" (Isaiah 26:3). Are you focused on the goal or on God?

TRUTH I WILL FOCUS ON TODAY

_____

_____

_____

_____

MY PRAYER

_____

_____

_____

_____

DAY 3

Scripture: **PROVERBS 18:14**

The human spirit can endure a sick body, but who can bear a crushed spirit?

DEVOTIONAL THOUGHT

When you have a broken leg, you can still hobble along. But when your heart is broken or your confidence shattered, you can barely move. As the writer of this proverb avers, a crushed spirit is the ultimate stop sign in a person's life. Setbacks in reaching a goal can pound the spirit. Staying the course seems as difficult as climbing a mountain.

Only God can revive a crushed, puréed spirit. He does it one step at a time. What small steps do you sense He is leading you to take?

TRUTH I WILL FOCUS ON TODAY

_____

_____

_____

_____

MY PRAYER

_____

_____

_____

_____

DAY 4

Scripture: GENESIS 33:13–14

But Jacob replied, "You can see, my lord, that some of the children are very young, and the flocks and herds have their young, too. If they are driven too hard, even for one day, all the animals could die. Please, my lord, go ahead of your servant. We will follow slowly, at a pace that is comfortable for the livestock and the children. I will meet you at Seir."

DEVOTIONAL THOUGHT

Although Jacob had the motive of putting some distance between himself and his brother, Esau, this passage reminds us to avoid exceeding our limitations. When we set a goal, we're sometimes tempted to think we can reach it faster if we double the pace or exceed the short-term goal. Instead of sticking to a 1300-calorie-a-day diet, we try to slash the calories to just 600 to 800 calories. Sadly, the risk of burnout increases.

During times like these, following wise advice is helpful. While we don't want to avoid challenging ourselves, we don't want to overdo it either. Who can you consult as you consider how to meet your goals?

TRUTH I WILL FOCUS ON TODAY

_____

_____

_____

_____

MY PRAYER

_____

_____

_____

_____

DAY 5

Scripture: PROVERBS 1:32

For simpletons turn away from me [wisdom]—to death. Fools are destroyed by their own complacency.

DEVOTIONAL THOUGHT

Complacency, like procrastination, is the great destroyer of lives. Sometimes we're fooled into believing that we know what we're doing. But as this proverb suggests, we need to admit our need for wisdom and to seek it. We're foolish if we ignore God's wisdom. It can't get much plainer than that!

Who or what is the voice of wisdom in your life right now? Perhaps a spouse has been telling you to avoid taking on too much too quickly. Maybe a friend has been trying to tell you something that you've ignored up till now. Sometimes the voice of wisdom comes unexpectedly. Are you listening?

TRUTH I WILL FOCUS ON TODAY

_____

_____

_____

_____

MY PRAYER

_____

_____

_____

_____

DAY 6

Scripture: MATTHEW 6:34

So don't worry about tomorrow, for tomorrow will bring its own worries. Today's trouble is enough for today.

DEVOTIONAL THOUGHT

How often have we mouthed Jesus' words from the Sermon on the Mount and yet failed to act on them? We get discouraged as we add up the weeks we have left before our goal is accomplished. We become overwhelmed by worrying about *how* we can accomplish the goal. Worry is as insidious as cancer. It eats away at us, sapping our life. That's why Jesus had so much to say about it.

What are the worries of tomorrow that you need to leave alone today? Consider spending some time in prayer, asking God for the strength to deposit all your worries with Him. "Don't borrow trouble" the old saying goes. You can never pay it back.

TRUTH I WILL FOCUS ON TODAY

_____

_____

_____

_____

MY PRAYER

_____

_____

_____

_____

DAY 7

Scripture: 1 CORINTHIANS 3:10–11

Because of God's grace to me, I have laid the foundation like an expert builder. Now others are building on it. But whoever is building on this foundation must be very careful. For no one can lay any foundation other than the one we already have—Jesus Christ.

DEVOTIONAL THOUGHT

To settle the "Paul versus Apollos" debate going on in the Corinthian church, Paul explained to the believers about the nature of his ministry to them—and upon whom it was built. Although he had laid the foundation for their faith, he could take no credit. It would come to nothing without God's grace and the work of Christ in their hearts. During Old Testament times, Solomon put it this way: "Unless the LORD builds a house, the work of the builders is wasted. Unless the LORD protects a city, guarding it with sentries will do no good" (Psalm 127:1).

When we work hard to accomplish our goals, we want some applause for our efforts. But how often do we thank God for sustaining us to meet those goals? If you haven't already thanked God, it's not too late.

TRUTH I WILL FOCUS ON TODAY

_____

_____

_____

_____

MY PRAYER

_____

_____

_____

_____

WEEKLY PROGRESS AND GOALS

❖ Current weight: _____

❖ Pounds lost this week: _____

NEW INSIGHTS

❖ About myself:

_____

_____

❖ From Scripture:

_____

_____

❖ About weight loss:

_____

_____

PLAN FOR NEXT WEEK

❖ Personal issue to focus on:

_____

_____

❖ Biblical truth to live out:

_____

_____

❖ Food to eliminate or restrict for the week:

_____

_____

❖ Exercise goals:

_____

_____

INTRODUCTION

May the Force be with you!" In the movie *Star Wars*, the idea of working with the "Force" is a consistent theme. Obi-Wan Kenobi, a main character, describes the Force as "an energy field created by all living things. It surrounds us, penetrates us, and binds the galaxy together." This energy field supposedly has a light side and dark side, both of which can be found inside humans, triggered by their emotions. Luke Skywalker and friends fight for the light side, while Darth Vader embodies the dark side. Yet at times the viewer sees the dark side in Luke and glimpses a bit of the light side even in Darth Vader.

Although the notion of a dualistic good/evil force is far from Christian theology, the Bible does say that all believers have a battle going on between our old sinful nature and our renewed life in the Christ. And the Bible makes it clear that we have a choice. We can allow the "light side" (God's Holy Spirit) to drive our motivations and emotions, or we can give in to the "dark side" (our sinful human nature) and fall back into old habits. What force, triggered by your emotions, drives you? There is always a choice.

VIDEO 12

Notes from video:

_____

_____

_____

_____

_____

_____

_____

_____

_____

_____

LIFL CONCEPT 12

IT IS NOT SO MUCH ABOUT THE FOOD WE EAT AS THE FORCES WITHIN US THAT DRIVE OUR EATING. NO DIET WILL HELP US RESOLVE THE EMOTIONAL TRIGGERS THAT CAUSE US TO OVEREAT.

Usually we have reasons for our actions. That is, something conscious or subconscious has urged, nudged, pushed, or pulled us to go a certain direction. We saw in previous sessions that resentments can cause us to explode in anger at an unsuspecting victim, and that bitterness and withholding forgiveness can keep us from moving forward. But other internal forces may be at work as well.

These driving forces may be easy to identify in other people: the classic Little League father who pushes his son, pressures the coach, and berates the umpire, hoping to relive his athletic glory days; the mother who dresses her little girl like a miniature adult and parades her through "beauty" pageants, hoping to affirm herself through her child; the woman working on her self-esteem issues; the man struggling with mid-life. But similar internal forces are at work within us as well—even though we may not see them (or may deny their existence).

Some of the internal forces are emotional triggers that move us toward less-than-healthy and sometimes destructive eating habits, such as overeating, binge eating and drinking, or satisfying that craving for sweets. We must identify those forces—the emotional triggers—so we can deal with them. If we don't, we won't be able to control or change our eating habits.

SCRIPTURE

1 CORINTHIANS 11:17–34

But in the following instructions, I cannot praise you. For it sounds as if more harm than good is done when you meet together. First, I hear that there are divisions among you when you meet as a church, and to some extent I believe it. But, of course, there must be divisions among you so that you who have God's approval will be recognized!

When you meet together, you are not really interested in the Lord's Supper. For some of you hurry to eat your own meal without sharing with others. As a result, some go hungry while others get drunk. What? Don't you have your own homes for eating and drinking? Or do you really want to disgrace God's church and shame the poor? What am I supposed to say? Do you want me to praise you? Well, I certainly will not praise you for this!

For I pass on to you what I received from the Lord himself. On the night when he was betrayed, the Lord Jesus took some bread and gave thanks to God for it. Then he broke it in pieces and said, "This is my body, which is given for you. Do this to remember me." In the same way, he took the cup of wine after supper, saying, "This cup is the new covenant between God and his people—an agreement confirmed with my blood. Do this to remember me as often as you drink it." For every time you eat this bread and drink this cup, you are announcing the Lord's death until he comes again.

So anyone who eats this bread or drinks this cup of the Lord unworthily is guilty of sinning against the body and blood of the Lord. That is why you should examine yourself before eating the bread and drinking the cup. For if you eat the bread or drink the cup without honoring the body of Christ, you are eating and drinking God's judgment upon yourself. That is why many of you are weak and sick and some have even died.

But if we would examine ourselves, we would not be judged by God in this way. Yet when we are judged by the Lord, we are being disciplined so that we will not be condemned along with the world.

So, my dear brothers and sisters, when you gather for the Lord's Supper, wait for each other. If you are really hungry, eat at home so you won't bring judgment upon yourselves when you meet together. I'll give you instructions about the other matters after I arrive.

This is one of the best-known passages about the Lord's Supper. But it also discusses our attitudes toward food. The way in which Christians share in Communion can give us a good idea of problems within the body of Christ. Paul's words to the Corinthian Christians about the Lord's Supper were meant to correct as much as they were meant to instruct. So we need to pay attention and listen carefully.

We probably know more about the Corinthian church's dirty laundry than any other church mentioned in the New Testament. By comparison, many churches today could take hope. Unfortunately, many of today's churches are also taking on some Corinthian characteristics—cliques, arguments, tolerance for blatant sin, and mixed-up priorities. Like the church at large today, the Corinthian Christians were under constant cultural pressure to conform, adjust, and ignore the teaching of Christ and the apostles.

One of the conflicts concerned food. This passage about the Lord's Supper concludes a long section that begins back at 1 Corinthians 8, where Paul refers to an issue he was asked to settle: "Now regarding your question about food that has been offered to idols. Yes, we know that 'we all have knowledge' about this issue. But while knowledge makes us feel important, it is love that strengthens the church" (1 Corinthians 8:1).

The use of animals and other food as offerings in worship had historical roots among the Jews as well as among the pagans. Remember Genesis 4, the key Bible passage for LIFL Concept Nine? It focused on the animal and food sacrifices Abel and Cain brought to God. In reading about the sacrificial system in the Old Testament, we learn that very little of the animals was actually burned on the altar. The meat left over from the sacrifice would feed the priests and often would be used in national celebrations as part of the thanksgiving buffet. The sacrifices of many fed all.

In Corinth, the pagan priests practiced a form of "recycling" animal sacrifices. It's quite possible that the worship ceremony primarily consisted of killing and bleeding the offered animals. What then to do with all the meat? It was sold in the marketplace.

These fine cuts of meat were certainly edible, but many Christians felt squeamish about consuming food that had been used in pagan ceremonies. It reminded them of their old way of living. Wasn't the meat spiritually tainted? This may be a difficult issue for us to identify with, since sacrificing animals isn't generally practiced in our culture. But we can understand their situation a bit more by imagining how we would feel if we were invited to go dumpster-diving behind a local steak restaurant in search of leftovers for a meal. Where our food had been and what it had been used for would make a difference then, even to us. Paul didn't settle the issue by declaring whether it was right or wrong to eat meat that had been offered to idols. But he did highlight the Christian rule that people are more important than food. Right and wrong doesn't have to do with what we eat but with how we treat ourselves and others by when, why, and how we eat.

Paul stated that while Christians have great freedom that extends even to our eating habits, it does not extend to the point that we can freely and deliberately offend other Christians. Some believers in Corinth felt offended by other believers who felt free to eat recycled meat. Other Christians were insisting that no one should infringe on their freedom in Christ to eat anything they wanted. Paul understood that eating is not a mindless consumption of fuel for living. Eating is a complex behavior that includes physical, psychological, emotional, and social elements. Paul was addressing the same underlying issues we find addressed in Concept Twelve: "It is not so much about the food we eat but the forces within us that drive our eating. No diet will help us resolve the emotional triggers that cause us to overeat."

Paul saw so much spiritual potential in the Corinthians, yet he also saw their fellowship unraveling through selfish interests. Individual appetites and fears were driving them, without consideration for others. Their worship was becoming dysfunctional.

In Paul's day, the Lord's Supper often was celebrated in the context of Christian love feasts—an early version of the church potluck meal. Early Christian churches included a cross-section of society; thus, a gathering in which everyone would bring food to share could result in a decent meal for many who would otherwise go hungry. But those who had enough, Paul discovered, were gorging themselves ahead of time, so they wouldn't risk getting less than they were used to eating. Instead of love feasts, the Corinthians were gathering for meals of leftovers. Some were already too full to eat anything while others went away hungry because of the meager table. As a result, the Lord's Supper was becoming a meaningless religious ritual rather than a time of spiritual clarity and reconnection with Christ's sacrificial death.

Paul insisted that self-examination is a key to personal and corporate spiritual health. The Communion table offers us a regular moment to reconsider how we're pursuing life. We must continue to acknowledge that we are sinners. We must recognize that we still need a Savior. As long as we live, we will continue to need His help with the ongoing effects of living in a fallen world.

At Communion we can practice Concept Two, using David's three-part prayer about sin (Psalm 19:12–14) to admit that we allow "emotional triggers" to drive destructive behaviors. We can benefit from Concept Twelve and ask God to help us identify those triggers and resolve the underlying issues. Christ is in this with us for the long haul. We need Him every day and every step of the way. That's why we take the bread and cup and remember His death until He comes again.

DISCUSSION QUESTIONS ABOUT SCRIPTURE

❖ What was the problem in Corinth regarding eating food that had been offered to idols?

_____

_____

_____

_____

❖ What problems does Paul address in this passage concerning their love feasts?

_____

_____

_____

_____

❖ What issues and emotional triggers lay behind the Corinthians' eating problems?

_____

_____

_____

_____

❖ How does Paul address those issues and emotional triggers?

_____

_____

_____

_____

❖ What does Communion mean? What is its purpose?

_____

_____

_____

_____

❖ How can remembering Christ's death help us lose it for life?

_____

_____

_____

_____

CASE STUDY

COREY

Love stinks sometimes. At least that was Corey's assessment. He was in love with Vicki. She turned him inside out with just a look. But when she ignored him, flirted with other guys, or broke up with him (as she had in the past), he just couldn't handle it.

Although Corey felt angry with Vicki when he wasn't with her, he found it difficult to express his anger. He didn't want to be like his dad, who was verbally abusive to his mom. So he took the anger out on himself by overindulging—drinking too much; eating way too much. Because of both, he had a sixty-pound weight gain to overcome.

But when Vicki apologized yet again for hurting him, all was right with the world. Corey easily slipped back into the routine of the low cholesterol diet his doctor assigned him. In fact, he even skipped some meals. Who needs food when you have love?

Now he was off his diet again. Vicki wanted to break up with him again. The donuts at work were starting to look mighty tempting.

YOUR TURN

❖ What is Corey's problem?

_____

_____

_____

_____

_____

❖ Why does he find it difficult to stick to his low cholesterol diet?

_____

_____

_____

_____

_____

❖ What emotional triggers affect Corey's eating habits and subsequent weight gain?

_____

_____

_____

_____

❖ What might Corey do to change this pattern?

_____

_____

_____

_____

AS A GROUP

❖ Besides love or lack of it, what other emotional triggers can cause a person to overeat?

_____

_____

_____

_____

❖ What can someone do to discover those triggers?

_____

_____

_____

_____

❖ How can we conquer them?

_____

_____

_____

_____

CHALLENGE

The first-century Corinthian believers found that past associations with paganism affected their love feasts. Corey's eating habits were determined more by his girlfriend's moods than by a conscious effort to control his weight. Emotional triggers can be as varied as human experience. Some people eat when they're excited or to celebrate. Others gorge when they're depressed. Some overindulge with food or drink (or worse) in certain situations or locations. And for many, a specific combination of people does the trick.

Our actions aren't _determined_ by the past or by present circumstances—so we shouldn't look for excuses for our poor choices. But memories, wounds, victories, and failures can conspire to push us in the wrong direction. So we need to identify those influential and powerful forces within us. Then we will be better prepared to deal with them, put them behind us, and move forward.

Consider the emotional factors that might be influencing your behavior. List your potential triggers. Ask someone who knows you and cares about you to help with this. Be sure to pray about this, too. Then give those past and present issues to God and take the next step toward your goal.

Daily Devotional Journal

DAY 1

Scripture: LAMENTATIONS 3:40

Instead, let us test and examine our ways. Let us turn back to the LORD.

DEVOTIONAL THOUGHT

In his agony over the destruction of Jerusalem and exile, the prophet Jeremiah expressed his people's need to return to the Lord. They'd blown it and were paying for their mistakes. The temptation for them was to believe that God had ceased to care for them.

Sometimes when we face a setback in our goal, the temptation is to remain off course. After all, backtracking can be difficult. It gets harder unless we first examine where we lost the trail in the first place. Are you "off the trail"? What do you need to do to get back?

TRUTH I WILL FOCUS ON TODAY

_____

_____

_____

_____

MY PRAYER

_____

_____

_____

_____

DAY 2

Scripture: 2 CORINTHIANS 13:5

Examine yourselves to see if your faith is genuine. Test yourselves. Surely you know that Jesus Christ is among you; if not, you have failed the test of genuine faith.

DEVOTIONAL THOUGHT

Instead of worrying about whether or not he spoke for Christ, Paul urged the believers in Corinth to examine themselves. In other words, were their motives Christlike? Did they rely on the Holy Spirit within them to recognize God's spokesperson? Or were they just trying to be critical?

Too often we judge other peoples' motives instead of examining our own. Or we focus on others' mistakes and use them as excuses for our lack of motivation. If we find one little glitch in someone's plan or advice, well, "obviously, he didn't know what he was talking about!"

"First get rid of the log in your own eye," Jesus advised in the Sermon on the Mount (Luke 6:42). God wants us to look within before looking out.

TRUTH I WILL FOCUS ON TODAY

_____

_____

_____

_____

MY PRAYER

_____

_____

_____

_____

DAY 3

Scripture: **PSALM 26:2**

Put me on trial, LORD, and cross-examine me. Test my motives and my heart.

DEVOTIONAL THOUGHT

David's bold prayer for God to examine his motives is a model of transparency. It allowed God carte blanche in every room in David's heart. He could test everything with His heavenly "white glove test."

We might wish to hide some of our motives from God—for example, our fears or jealousies or resentments. We fear the spotlight of God's truth. But God loves you. Do you believe that? As you pray David's prayer, allow Him to have an all-access pass into your heart motives.

TRUTH I WILL FOCUS ON TODAY

_____

_____

_____

_____

MY PRAYER

_____

_____

_____

_____

DAY 4

Scripture: 1 JOHN 3:20

Even if we feel guilty, God is greater than our feelings, and he knows everything.

DEVOTIONAL THOUGHT

When we fail, we're the first to condemn ourselves. Guilt consumes us and causes us to fear trying again. That's why the apostle John's message is so comforting. It asserts that God is greater than the weight of guilt we may feel! He knows our strengths and weaknesses better than we know them.

Feeling buried under a load of guilt? God is greater than any load of guilt. Are you willing to trust Him?

TRUTH I WILL FOCUS ON TODAY

_____

_____

_____

_____

MY PRAYER

_____

_____

_____

_____

DAY 5

Scripture: PSALM 4:4

Don't sin by letting anger control you. Think about it overnight and remain silent.

DEVOTIONAL THOUGHT

What positive skills or habits have you mastered? A sport? Sticking to your diet? How about controlling anger? Many of us have the mistaken belief that we have our anger under control. That belief lasts until someone cuts us off in traffic or humiliates us in public.

In Ephesians 4:26, Paul echoes David's words: " 'Don't sin by letting anger gain control over you.' Don't let the sun go down while you are still angry." This verse stresses the need to avoid holding a grudge or letting it lead to something worse.

Feeling angry? Don't hold on to it. Confront it instead, because this emotion can trigger a host of problems.

TRUTH I WILL FOCUS ON TODAY

_____

_____

_____

_____

MY PRAYER

_____

_____

_____

_____

DAY 6

Scripture: GALATIANS 5:17

The sinful nature wants to do evil, which is just the opposite of what the Spirit wants. And the Spirit gives us desires that are the opposite of what the sinful nature desires. These two forces are constantly fighting each other, so you are not free to carry out your good intentions.

DEVOTIONAL THOUGHT

The apostle Paul wrote out of his awareness of human nature. Our good intentions war with our desire to sin. Sometimes we lose a skirmish when our emotions get in the way. If we're angry or depressed, we might eat more or feel like giving up.

Paul expressed the same sentiment in another way: "I want to do what is good, but I don't. I don't want to do what is wrong, but I do it anyway. But if I do what I don't want to do, I am not really the one doing wrong; it is sin living in me that does it" (Romans 7:19–20). So what's the solution? "There is no condemnation for those who belong to Christ Jesus. And because you belong to him, the power of the life-giving Spirit has freed you from the power of sin that leads to death" (Romans 8:1–2).

Forces may be at war within us, but the Holy Spirit frees us from our bent toward sin. Thanks be to God!

TRUTH I WILL FOCUS ON TODAY

_____

_____

_____

_____

MY PRAYER

_____

_____

_____

_____

DAY 7

Scripture: ROMANS 8:6

So letting your sinful nature control your mind leads to death. But letting the Spirit control your mind leads to life and peace.

DEVOTIONAL THOUGHT

We've seen the effects of living according to one's basest desires. The evening news is full of stories where the innocent and not-so-innocent wind up dead because of them. That's why some of the strongest warnings in the Bible concern the flesh and the effect our sinful desires have on the mind.

Winning the battle of the mind is the first victory in the battle of the bulge. If we live our lives by our own rules, we will lose. The solution, according to Paul, is to live by the Spirit's control.

Many centuries ago David had this advice for those who would ignore God's direction: "Do not be like a senseless horse or mule that needs a bit and bridle to keep it under control" (Psalm 32:9). Joyfully submit to God's way and let His Spirit lead you.

TRUTH I WILL FOCUS ON TODAY

_____

_____

_____

_____

MY PRAYER

_____

_____

_____

_____

WEEKLY PROGRESS AND GOALS

❖ Current weight: _____

❖ Pounds lost this week: _____

NEW INSIGHTS

❖ About myself:

_____

_____

❖ From Scripture:

_____

_____

❖ About weight loss:

_____

_____

PLAN FOR NEXT WEEK

❖ Personal issue to focus on:

_____

_____

❖ Biblical truth to live out:

_____

_____

❖ Food to eliminate or restrict for the week:

_____

_____

❖ Exercise goals:

_____

_____

INTRODUCTION

Perfect. We hear the term all the time. "That dress fits you perfectly." "That shot was perfect." To be *perfect* means to be without any flaws or imperfections. So was the dress or golf shot perfect? Hardly.

Yet society seems to imply that we need to be perfect. We won't be accepted until we look hip and exude happiness. At least that's how the airbrushed models look. And being perfect is what it will take to find love, a rewarding career, and a meaningful life. So we think that we have to have it all together. Our lives must be perfect or we won't be loved. Thus, many people work late hours, live in mansions, or get liposuction because they want acceptance and love.

God's love is different. He loves us just the way we are, no matter what. This means that nothing can change how much God loves us. And He loves us completely, imperfections and all. We don't have to dress up, act a certain way, or put on a perfect front to impress Him or to earn His acceptance. His love will never change.

The problem with trying to be perfect is that we will always fail. And the more we strive to be perfect, the more we will fall short of it. Your goal shouldn't be to obtain a perfect image but to glorify God and serve Him more fully. Let that motivate you.

VIDEO 13

Notes from video:

_____

_____

_____

_____

_____

_____

_____

_____

_____

_____

_____

LIFL CONCEPT 13

GOD WON'T LOVE YOU MORE IF YOU LOSE WEIGHT. BUT HE CAN USE YOU MORE EFFECTIVELY THROUGHOUT A LONGER LIFE IF YOU MAKE CHANGES THAT RESULT IN BEING ABLE TO LIVE CONSISTENTLY AT THE WEIGHT THAT IS BEST FOR YOU.

In a TV sit-com a couple of decades ago, a main character would often say, "God will get you for this!" The meaning was clear: *God is waiting for us to mess up, and when we do, wham! He punishes us.* It's a common misconception of God. And it usually comes with another thought on the flipside: *When we do good, God will reward us. In fact, He'll love us more!* This view of God may keep some people from doing wrong, but it certainly has become a burden. That's because we'll never be good enough. No one's perfect, so with this view of God, we'll always harbor doubts about His love for us.

The truth? God loves us—period. His love cannot be earned; it's a gift, freely given. And if we ever doubt that, remember what Jesus did on the cross (see John 3:16).

Does that mean we should stop working to be better and do better? Of course not. But our reason should be that we can serve Him better and more fully. That makes sense, right? A person who lives longer will be able to serve God longer. A healthy person will be able to use his or her strength and energy to serve Him. So don't worry about being perfect. Do be concerned, however, about being your best—for His sake.

SCRIPTURE

EPHESIANS 3:17–19

Then Christ will make his home in your hearts as you trust in him. Your roots will grow down into God's love and keep you strong. And may you have the power to understand, as all God's people should, how wide, how long, how high, and how deep his love is. May you experience the love of Christ, though it is too great to understand fully. Then you will be made complete with all the fullness of life and power that comes from God.

After living with Concept Twelve for a week, we may be thinking that being trigger-happy emotionally is not a good thing. We were reminded about the ongoing nature of our struggle with sin, and that the concepts in LIFL are not instant, one-time solutions to our deepest issues in life. These Concepts do allow us to deal meaningfully with those issues by giving us resources for the journey. Every Concept is a reminder of our need for God's help.

Concept Thirteen allows us to think carefully about perhaps the central emotional trigger that motivates our actions in almost every situation—our longing for love. We may confuse that longing with other "hungers," but our efforts to satisfy those other hungers don't touch our persistent need for love. Even our relationship with God can be profoundly affected if we conclude that God's love is given to us based on performance. That error creates a false emotional trigger that can create havoc in us.

Affirming that God loves the *world* takes little risk. We have John 3:16 to back us up: "For God loved the world so much that he gave his one and only Son, so that everyone who believes in him will not perish but have eternal life." But our longing for love may lead us to think that even a love as great as God's, subdivided to as many people as there are in the world, doesn't leave much love for any one person. Combine this idea with the conditional love from others who have doled out acceptance based on our performance, and it's easy to go through life thinking that love is earned. We can even assume that we must earn God's love.

But God's love isn't a commodity on the stock market. God's love for us doesn't rise or fall depending on how many shares we own, bought by our good works. And the value of God's love doesn't change depending on worldwide demand. God's love is not a large version of anything on earth. At best, love at the human level is a dim, mirror image of that character trait of God that escapes all limitations and boundaries—His love.

One of the best descriptions of what it means to know God's love can be found in Ephesians 3:16–21. This passage is Paul's prayer for the Ephesian believers. By extension, that prayer applies to us as believers as well. The point of the prayer is to connect us with God's boundless love. Understanding and experiencing the height, depth, length, and width of God's love doesn't mean that we can somehow measure it. Instead, it will overwhelm us by realizing that God's love is immeasurable!

Our attempts to earn or deserve more love from God are sad and empty because we carry them out in the face of God's boundless love. This misunderstanding turns around the order of life, and no amount of frantic effort on our part can straighten it out again. If our relationship with God in any way begins or relies on us, we will always feel as though we're trying to catch up to something that is leaving us behind. But if our relationship with God begins with His unchanging, unconditional, fully-operational-when-we-are-at-our-very-worst kind of love, well, that changes the meaning of everything we do! We are forever responding to His great love. If God's love is constant, then life is not about earning more or deserving more but about thanking more and enjoying more!

Almost instinctively we know that life seems easier to face when we know that we are loved. But if we've got the order of life turned around, we are always trying to be loved so that life will get easier, rather than centering on the fact that God loves us and letting life flow out of that great discovery! Every positive decision in life, from losing weight to speaking the truth, takes on renewed possibilities in the atmosphere of God's love. But picturing ourselves outside God's love, desperately trying to get *in,* means we've turned around the order of life.

If what you just read switched on a light in your soul, God's Spirit is speaking to you. God is still answering Paul's ancient prayer today. People are still discovering that God takes lives that are turned the wrong way and lovingly turns them the right way. God loves you the same when you are going either way. But when you are thinking and living in the freedom of His love, your awareness of His boundless love will become increasingly clear. The challenges won't suddenly become easy or life trouble-free. Sometimes, just the opposite occurs. But the light of God's love makes even the "impossible" look different.

God's love is an energizing power. The confidence in Paul's prayer is infectious—let it infect you! "Now all glory to God, who is able, through his mighty power at work within us, to accomplish infinitely more than we might ask or think" (Ephesians 3:20). Set aside for a moment all the things you wish you could accomplish, all the goals you hardly dare to whisper, and begin to think of what might happen as a result of God's love and power flowing through you. Always start with God rather than yourself and you'll go a lot farther than you ever expected!

DISCUSSION QUESTIONS ABOUT SCRIPTURE

❖ What evidence do you see in others of the universal longing for love? How about in yourself?

_____

_____

_____

_____

_____

❖ How might this longing affect a person's understanding of God's love?

_____

_____

_____

_____

❖ When did you learn about God's love for you?

_____

_____

_____

_____

_____

_____

❖ What examples can you give of the "height, depth, length, width" of God's love that you have experienced?

_____

_____

_____

_____

_____

_____

❖ Why might someone think that he or she has to *earn* God's love? How could this misunderstanding affect that person's ability to lose weight?

_____

_____

_____

_____

_____

_____

❖ How do you know that God loves each person, including *you*, unconditionally?

_____

_____

_____

_____

_____

❖ How can knowing this truth affect a person's ability to lose weight?

_____

_____

_____

_____

_____

CASE STUDY

RACHEL

Rachel peered at herself in the mirror, thinking of how people used to say that she looked a lot like Jennifer Aniston, except, well, heavier. Now that she'd lost thirty pounds, people were starting to say the same words without the "heavier" qualifier.

She smoothed down the black dress. Although she'd reached her goal weight, she could still see a little bit of a midriff bulge. *Maybe I can lose another twenty.*

"Honey, you look great," her husband Jake said warmly.

Rachel's expression showed her disagreement. "Instead of going to the steak place tonight, can we go to the salad place?"

Jake looked momentarily confused. "Why? I thought you wanted to go there to celebrate reaching your goal weight."

"I think I need to lose at least twenty more pounds."

"And look like a stick?! C'mon, Rach! You look great now!"

But Rachel wasn't listening. With another twenty pounds gone, she'd look exactly like Jennifer and like that model she saw on the cover of *Vogue*. Yes. Then life would be perfect.

YOUR TURN

❖ What do you think motivated Rachel to try to lose weight in the first place?

_____

_____

_____

_____

_____

❖ Why did she think that she had to lose more?

_____

_____

_____

_____

_____

_____

❖ Why didn't Rachel hear Jake's compliments and concerns?

_____

_____

_____

_____

_____

_____

❖ When do you think Rachel will be satisfied with her weight and look?

_____

_____

_____

_____

_____

_____

AS A GROUP

❖ How real are the pictures of models on magazine covers and in ads?

_____

_____

_____

_____

_____

❖ Why do we think we should look like them? Why do we try?

_____

_____

_____

_____

_____

❖ Why do people think others will like or love them more if they're "perfect"? How might this carry over into how we think about God?

_____

_____

_____

_____

_____

❖ How should knowing that God loves us unconditionally affect the way we live?

_____

_____

_____

_____

_____

CHALLENGE

No one wants to be left out, alone, or on the outside looking in. Everyone wants to be included, accepted, and welcomed. To love and be loved is a basic human need. And because we're often driven by this powerful emotional motive, we may take our lives in unusual directions. Consider what a couple in love will do for each other, the sacrifices a parent will make for a child, the selfless service of a friend for a friend, and our overwhelming grief at the loss of a loved one. Love is powerful.

Nothing is more powerful and motivating than the love of God. And, amazingly, His love is perfect, undeserved, freely given, and everlasting. Jesus died for us *totally undeserving sinners* (Romans 5:8). We could never earn God's love, and nothing we can do will make Him love us more. And get this: *we can never be lost to God's love* (Romans 8:38–39).

So how does that make you feel? Live in the light of God's love!

DAILY DEVOTIONAL JOURNAL

DAY 1

Scripture: GALATIANS 2:19

For when I tried to keep the law, it condemned me. So I died to the law—I stopped trying to meet all its requirements—so that I might live for God.

DEVOTIONAL THOUGHT

Even Paul—the man who wrote most of the New Testament—could not live up to the perfect standards of the law of Moses. The law could only show how far off-course people were. It emphasized the need for a Savior, whose perfect life fulfilled the law.

Sometimes we have a perfectionist mentality about life. We try to perfectly follow the rules and expect others to adhere to them as well. And we think that God will love us more and give us more if we do more for Him. In our quest for perfection, we take an unexpected detour into legalism. If we're not careful, a critical spirit is the result of the journey. Are you finding yourself in that territory? Like Paul, are you willing to "die to the law"?

TRUTH I WILL FOCUS ON TODAY

_____

_____

_____

_____

MY PRAYER

_____

_____

_____

_____

DAY 2

Scripture: 1 CORINTHIANS 8:8

It's true that we can't win God's approval by what we eat. We don't lose anything if we don't eat it, and we don't gain anything if we do.

DEVOTIONAL THOUGHT

Concerning eating meat offered to idols (is it allowable or not allowable), Paul offered words of freedom for those who feared doing the wrong thing. For those caught in the trap of legalism, he offered a reminder of what counts or does not count with God.

What counts with God? First Corinthians 8:6 says it all: "There is only one Lord, Jesus Christ, through whom God made everything and through whom we have been given life." Knowing the Lord—the One who truly *is* perfect—counts with God.

TRUTH I WILL FOCUS ON TODAY

_____

_____

_____

_____

MY PRAYER

_____

_____

_____

_____

DAY 3

Scripture: 1 JOHN 4:9–12

God showed how much he loved us by sending his one and only Son into the world so that we might have eternal life through him. This is real love—not that we loved God, but that he loved us and sent his Son as a sacrifice to take away our sins. Dear friends, since God loved us that much, we surely ought to love each other. No one has ever seen God. But if we love each other, God lives in us, and his love is brought to full expression in us.

DEVOTIONAL THOUGHT

Ever search for the perfect solution to a problem? We may consciously or subconsciously search for the "right" answer to life's questions and issues. Some problems have multiple-choice answers. But the problem of sin has only one answer, only one perfect choice: Jesus' death. Internalizing God's sacrificial love frees us to love others.

This sacrificial love causes us to see others in a new light. We focus less on imperfections and more on grace. Is that your way of looking at others?

TRUTH I WILL FOCUS ON TODAY

_____

_____

_____

_____

MY PRAYER

_____

_____

_____

_____

DAY 4

Scripture: ROMANS 3:20

For no one can ever be made right with God by doing what the law commands. The law simply shows us how sinful we are.

DEVOTIONAL THOUGHT

When we were kids, our parents might have used a yardstick or some other measuring device to gauge our height. Perhaps they drew a line on the wall each year as a marker.

The Law served as a marker as well. Sadly, it showed how far from God people were, as Paul explained to the believers in Rome. Instead of being a cause for discouragement, this is good news. Sure, we can't ever "get it perfectly right" with God. But we don't have to, thanks to Jesus. He's the only one who ever "got it right." Trusting Him makes us right with God.

In what ways are you trying to get it perfectly right these days? Perhaps you're discouraged over trying and failing to be letter-perfect in following a diet or living up to a standard others seem to have. What do you need to let go of?

TRUTH I WILL FOCUS ON TODAY

_____

_____

_____

MY PRAYER

_____

_____

_____

_____

DAY 5

Scripture: **ROMANS 14:17–18**

For the Kingdom of God is not a matter of what we eat or drink, but of living a life of goodness and peace and joy in the Holy Spirit. If you serve Christ with this attitude, you will please God, and others will approve of you, too.

DEVOTIONAL THOUGHT

Once again, Paul addresses the issue of food, this time to answer any questions Jewish and Gentile believers might have due to their differing lifestyles (kosher versus nonkosher foods; food or wine offered to idols, and so forth). Paul's goal was to quell legalistic attitudes about food and criticism of fellow believers. Instead of nitpicking, he reminded the believers of what they could have in abundance: goodness, peace, and joy—some of the fruit of the Holy Spirit.

When we're dieting, we get used to watching every calorie and narrowing the field of what's allowable. But this watchful state sometimes extends toward others as we monitor their food intake or other aspects of their lifestyles. "Are you sure you want to eat that popcorn? Haven't you had enough fat this week?" or "Should Christians watch that movie?" While nothing's wrong with being careful, we walk a fine line between concern and legalism.

Today, consider the fact that you can have all the goodness, peace, and joy you want. Revel in it. Then pass it on.

TRUTH I WILL FOCUS ON TODAY

_____

_____

_____

_____

MY PRAYER

_____

_____

_____

_____

DAY 6

Scripture: ROMANS 8:35

Can anything ever separate us from Christ's love? Does it mean he no longer loves us if we have trouble or calamity, or are persecuted, or hungry, or destitute, or in danger, or threatened with death?

DEVOTIONAL THOUGHT

"God seems so far away." Have you ever thought that? Perhaps during a crisis or a setback you've wondered whether God suddenly stopped caring or ever cared in the first place. Paul's words of assurance are a way of answering no to the question, "Has God stopped loving me because I'm suffering now?"

This assurance also goes with the issue of perfection. Let's face it—we're often conditional in our love for each other. "I'll love you as long as you _____"—fill in the blank with the love language action or standard of your choice. Sometimes these conditions come from the hurts inflicted by others. Perhaps a spouse rejected us when we put on the pounds. We long for unconditional love—love for us *despite* our weaknesses. That's the kind of love Jesus has for you. Meditate on that this week.

TRUTH I WILL FOCUS ON TODAY

_____

_____

_____

_____

MY PRAYER

_____

_____

_____

_____

DAY 7

Scripture: EPHESIANS 5:2

Live a life filled with love, following the example of Christ. He loved us and offered himself as a sacrifice for us, a pleasing aroma to God.

DEVOTIONAL THOUGHT

Think about the aromas that perk up your spirit. How about the aroma of that first cup of coffee in the morning? Or maybe it is your wife or girlfriend's perfume or that new car smell. Here, the sacrificial death of Christ is described as the ultimate "pleasing aroma." His death was more fragrant to God than the incense burning in the temple. It absolutely riveted God's attention.

What is the "aroma" of your life? A critical spirit has a way of diluting the pleasing aroma of a life, just as the scent of gasoline dilutes the "new car" smell of a vehicle. Need an aroma check? Consider Paul's advice. "Live a life filled with love." What actions show that love is your aroma?

TRUTH I WILL FOCUS ON TODAY

_____

_____

_____

_____

MY PRAYER

_____

_____

_____

_____

WEEKLY PROGRESS AND GOALS

❖ Current weight: _____

❖ Pounds lost this week: _____

NEW INSIGHTS

❖ About myself:

_____

_____

❖ From Scripture:

_____

_____

❖ About weight loss:

_____

_____

PLAN FOR NEXT WEEK

❖ Personal issue to focus on:

_____

_____

❖ Biblical truth to live out:

_____

_____

❖ Food to eliminate or restrict for the week:

_____

_____

❖ Exercise goals:

_____

_____

INTRODUCTION

Please mom, puh-lease!!" begged Tommy. "Please can I have just one cookie?"

"I told you already—no cookies until after dinner," his mom patiently replied.

With shoulders slumped and feet dragging, Tommy dramatically left the room. His mom couldn't keep herself from shaking her head and smiling. Checking the casserole in the oven, she wiped her hands on her apron and retreated to the living room.

A few minutes later, she heard tiny feet tiptoe into the kitchen. She quietly walked to the entrance and watched. Tommy, looking over his shoulder, cautiously climbed on a chair and then onto the counter to the cookie jar, opened it, and stuck in his hand. Quick—what do you think Tommy's mom is thinking? Is she upset? Perhaps—certainly disappointed. He is blatantly disobeying her, so she will have to discipline him. But does Mom love Tommy any less?

"Tommy, what are you doing? Didn't I tell you no? Please get down from the counter and come over here!"

Tommy slowly put the lid down, climbed off the chair, and shuffled toward his mom, focused on the floor. He looked up at her with big brown eyes brimming with tears, waiting to receive his deserved punishment. Now—what is Tommy thinking? He may be thinking (especially if he is a sensitive child), *I didn't obey. Now Mom hates me, and she'll never love me again.*

Was Tommy's offense serious? Of course—he disobeyed his mom. But that doesn't mean she loves him any less. It's the same with us and God. We make mistakes and fail, but does God love us any less? No. God doesn't always approve of our actions—and discipline may be in order—but His love isn't determined by what we do. He continues to love us, even in our disobedience.

VIDEO 14

Notes from video:

_____

_____

_____

_____

_____

_____

LIFL CONCEPT 14

WHEN YOU STUMBLE AND RELAPSE BACK INTO OLD UNHEALTHY PATTERNS, YOU MAY LOVE YOURSELF LESS, BUT GOD DOES NOT LOVE YOU LESS, AND YOU CAN DO NOTHING TO MAKE HIM LOVE YOU MORE.

We hit this concept last session when we discussed the fact that God's love for us is not contingent on our good deeds or actions. He accepts us as we are and loves us unconditionally. This shouldn't lead to laziness or disobedience. In reality, the more we understand God's love for us, the more we should be motivated to live His way and to serve Him. We also discussed in the last session that improving ourselves and living the right way can give us more opportunities to do just that.

So the discussion continues. In this session, we are considering how we will feel and react when we experience setbacks—when we stumble, fall, or relapse. We shouldn't expect to fall, but being human and, thus, imperfect, we can expect bumps in the road as we journey toward our goal. When we hit those bumps and potholes, we should remember that God still loves us and that He stands at the door of our lives, like Tommy's loving mother pictured above, watching, waiting, and encouraging us to make the necessary adjustments and move on.

SCRIPTURE

2 CORINTHIANS 4:7–18

We now have this light shining in our hearts, but we ourselves are like fragile clay jars containing this great treasure. This makes it clear that our great power is from God, not from ourselves.

We are pressed on every side by troubles, but we are not crushed. We are perplexed, but not driven to despair. We are hunted down, but never abandoned by God. We get knocked down, but we are not destroyed. Through suffering, our bodies continue to share in the death of Jesus so that the life of Jesus may also be seen in our bodies.

Yes, we live under constant danger of death because we serve Jesus, so that the life of Jesus will be evident in our dying bodies. So we live in the face of death, but this has resulted in eternal life for you.

But we continue to preach because we have the same kind of faith the psalmist had when he said, "I believed in God, so I spoke." We know that God, who raised the Lord Jesus, will also raise us with Jesus and present us to himself together with you. All of this is for your benefit. And as God's grace reaches more and more people, there will be great thanksgiving and God will receive more and more glory.

That is why we never give up. Though our bodies are dying, our spirits are being renewed every day. For our present troubles are small and won't last very long. Yet they produce for us a glory that vastly outweighs them and will last forever! So we don't look at the troubles we can see now; rather, we fix our gaze on things that cannot be seen. For the things we see now will soon be gone, but the things we cannot see will last forever.

Face it—the Bible treats us like dirt. We open Genesis and discover we were fashioned from mud (Genesis 2:7). Job reminds us that we are dust (Job 10:9). Take out the water that makes up the greatest percentage of our physical bodies, and we easily blow away in the wind. God reminds us in Isaiah and Jeremiah that He's the potter and we're the clay (Isaiah 29:16; Jeremiah 18:3–6). In one of His parables, Jesus explains that our hearts can resemble one of four kinds of dirt (Matthew 13:1–23). Now we come to a passage in which Paul admits that we're "fragile clay jars containing this great treasure." No wonder we feel so vulnerable, unstable, and breakable. We're cracked pots!

To be more precise, we are like *living* clay. As life's wheel spins us and we yield to surrounding pressures, sometimes we take on unexpected shapes. Given our identity, Concept Fourteen comes as no surprise: "When you stumble and relapse back into old unhealthy patterns, you may love yourself less, but God does not love you less and there is nothing you can do to make him love you more." We've had enough exposure to these concepts by now that we may be reading them haphazardly. But missing the very first word in Concept Fourteen will set us up for disappointment: *when. When* you stumble, not *if* you stumble. In order to honor the ongoing truth of Concept Two ("The biggest challenge is seeing the reality in our lives and telling ourselves the truth."), we must acknowledge that at every turn we will fall short of perfection both in planning and executing life. It's what living clay does. If we were perfect, we wouldn't be clay.

So the question becomes, how can we live as God's clay? How can we acknowledge Him as our Potter and remain moldable in His hands? This passage from 2 Corinthians gives priceless instruction. First, the emphasis is never on the container but always on the contents. When Christ is in us, we contain a "great treasure" (verse 7). Our flaws are painfully obvious—the world sees them. We may hide some of these flaws and not be aware of others, but plenty of unmistakable flaws will always be obvious for others to see. Paul's picture in these verses describes us as pots that have been glued back together multiple times by loving hands. But we're never "all we're cracked up to be." We may not like this self-portrait, but Paul thinks it has two distinct advantages: First, it's a true picture; second, it allows the "great treasure" we hold to be seen more clearly. When people look at our lives, we want them to run to Christ because of the amazing things He has done for cracked pots like us!

So how do we live as God's clay? Paul tells us we may run into four types of potentially shattering experiences that will affect us painfully, but that God can use effectively, "so that the life of Jesus may also be seen in our bodies." These jarring experiences include:

❖ "Pressing" experiences (verse 8) that come from troubles. These external pressures can make us feel like we are about to implode. If we were hollow clay containers, we wouldn't stand a chance. But to the degree that we allow the presence of Christ's Spirit to fill us, we can stand up to any pressure because the power of resistance comes from within us and is not "ours."

❖ "Perplexing" experiences (verse 8) that come from unexpected sources of pressure. Maybe a person we trust put expectations on us, making us perplexed. Areas of life that have been under control suddenly turn chaotic. The problems are familiar but unexpected—perplexing! Areas of life are never quite under control, and their wildness mocks and perplexes us. Those in Christ have these experiences and are faced with the choice every person faces: taking the way of despair and crumbling into clay shards, or taking the way of hope in Christ and relying on His power to go on.

❖ "Hunted" experiences (verse 9) that come from feeling targeted by life's trials. You've probably noticed a subtle sequence here. Even when we have responded to pressures and perplexing circumstances, we may then find ourselves struggling with that sense of unfairness we touched on in Concept Nine. We begin to think we're in the crosshairs of trouble. Fatigue and self-pity may start a chorus of whining that threatens to hit just the right pitch to shatter us. In those awful moments, Paul tells us, we are "never abandoned by God." As overwhelming as these challenges can be, we can be tempted to shout from our troubles as Jesus did, "My God, my God, why have you forsaken me?" (Mark 15:34) But we must remember that Jesus shouted those words so that we would never have to shout them. God abandoned Jesus to our sins so that He would never have to abandon us to them! God says to you what He said to Joshua, "I will never leave you or abandon you" (Joshua 1:5).

❖ "Knocked down" experiences (verse 9) that come from being pulled down by life. Sometimes we fall down; sometimes we get pushed. We think we're doing fine and the next moment we're flat on our faces, with no clue as to what happened. We're down but we're not out. Paul tells us, "We are not destroyed."

Paul goes on to say that all these are simply legs of the journey on the way to eternity. Eventually we will realize that these "present troubles are small and won't last very long. Yet they produce for us a glory that vastly outweighs them and will last forever!" (verse 17). They appear overwhelming because they are in our faces. Seen from eternity, they will be as nothing. For now, however, though we are painfully aware of our fragile nature as pottery, we choose to "fix our gaze on things that cannot be seen" (verse 18)—Christ's priceless presence in us. And we trust that others will somehow see Christ in us!

DISCUSSION QUESTIONS ABOUT SCRIPTURE

❖ Why does Paul use the picture of "fragile clay jars" to describe us? When, recently, have you felt like that?

_____

_____

_____

_____

_____

❖ What is "living" clay? Why is that a good description of us?

_____

_____

_____

_____

❖ What kinds of conditions or factors tend to push us out of shape? Which ones threaten to shatter us?

_____

_____

_____

_____

❖ What examples can you give of "perplexing" experiences?

_____

_____

_____

_____

❖ When have you felt "hunted"? How about "knocked down"?

_____

_____

_____

_____

❖ Why do these troubles often seem overwhelming?

_____

_____

_____

_____

❖ How do you feel about being a "cracked pot" in light of what Christ has done for you and in light of eternity? How does that knowledge affect how you live?

_____

_____

_____

_____

CASE STUDY

DEVLIN

"Dev! What happened to you?"

Devlin was used to those words spoken in a positive and a negative tone. A sixty-pound weight gain over a five-year period had that effect on people.

His wife, Bev, had begged him to lose weight, reminding him of the way he was when they were dating. "I want you around to see our daughter grow up," she had remarked.

Devlin had worked hard to lose twenty pounds. Now the scale was turning back toward the red zone. He couldn't help it. Work was stressful. So many clients to please. And his daughter Lindsay's private school tuition wasn't getting any lower. During the holidays there was so much food at work, so much temptation.

"Dev, are you're cheating on your diet?" his wife asked with folded arms.

He could see the look of disappointment in her eyes. "Of course not," he said, knowing that she knew he was lying.

YOUR TURN

❖ Why had Devlin decided to lose weight?

_____

_____

_____

_____

❖ Why is he struggling with that right now?

_____

_____

_____

_____

_____

❖ Why did Devlin lie to Bev?

_____

_____

_____

_____

_____

❖ How might this become a vicious and destructive cycle?

_____

_____

_____

_____

_____

❖ What will it take to get Dev back on track?

_____

_____

_____

_____

AS A GROUP

❖ What causes people to relapse into unhealthy lifestyle patterns?

_____

_____

_____

_____

❖ What daily reminders do we have that we are "fragile clay jars"?

_____

_____

_____

_____

❖ When we stumble and fall (or get cracked, as with clay), what can we do to get up and back on track?

_____

_____

_____

_____

❖ How does knowing that God loves us unconditionally help?

_____

_____

_____

_____

CHALLENGE

Have you stumbled lately? Of course you have. Everyone does. But stumbling or relapsing is only a problem if we stay down or if we quit the race entirely. And in this race, we should remember all those in the stands who are cheering us on—family, friends, and God Himself. They want us to finish well.

We took a close look at another helpful picture earlier—clay and the molding process. In this analogy, God is the potter, and we are His pots. We're fragile, easily misshapen or cracked by pressures and circumstances; but God can and will make us new. He promises that we won't be destroyed.

So don't let your setbacks set you back. Don't allow your let downs to get you down. Instead, remember God's unfailing and unconditional love. Ask for His power and direction, and move ahead.

DAILY DEVOTIONAL JOURNAL

DAY 1

Scripture: PSALM 86:5

O LORD, you are so good, so ready to forgive, so full of unfailing love for all who ask for your help.

DEVOTIONAL THOUGHT

"You blew it!" Words like this conjure up feelings of condemnation. *Who could ever love someone so imperfect?* we think. King David, who certainly knew what it felt like to fail (see 2 Samuel 11–12), decided not to focus on his cracked-clay life. He turned his eyes toward God. God's love and forgiveness were the perfect antidote—a healing sight for sore eyes that were weary of the view of his imperfect self.

When you've had it up to here with the *so* statements you hear in life ("You're so lazy"; "You're so pathetic"; "I'm so over you"; "That's why you're so fat."), why not trade them in for the truth of God? He's "so good, so ready to forgive, so full of unfailing love." Best of all, He's so in love with you.

TRUTH I WILL FOCUS ON TODAY

_____

_____

_____

_____

MY PRAYER

_____

_____

_____

_____

DAY 2

Scripture: **PSALM 31:7**

I will be glad and rejoice in your unfailing love, for you have seen my troubles, and you care about the anguish of my soul.

DEVOTIONAL THOUGHT

At times we may think no one understands our pain. We feel as brittle as a thin layer of ice on a window—one touch in the right place and we crumble. But God sees and knows all about us, as David writes in this psalm. This truth could cause us fear, but its purpose is not to punish us but to comfort us. God sees and knows all about you. He cares "about the anguish of my soul"—about the thoughts and feelings we're reluctant to reveal to anyone else. Doesn't the One who can see the anguish of your soul deserve your trust?

TRUTH I WILL FOCUS ON TODAY

_____

_____

_____

_____

MY PRAYER

_____

_____

_____

_____

DAY 3

Scripture: ISAIAH 43:2–3A

When you go through deep waters, I will be with you. When you go through rivers of difficulty, you will not drown. When you walk through the fire of oppression, you will not be burned up; the flames will not consume you. For I am the LORD, your God, the Holy One of Israel, your Savior.

DEVOTIONAL THOUGHT

Sometimes life feels like the deep end of the pool. You can't stand up in it; it's way over your head. In this passage from the prophet Isaiah, we are reminded that we, too, will find the promise of God's presence in life's overwhelming, most painful moments. During those times when we feel most helpless and vulnerable—as raw as an open wound—He is with us.

Instead of feeling overwhelmed or defeated, we can accept God's "CPR"—His power to overcome any adversity. In need of spiritual CPR? You only have to say one word: "Help."

TRUTH I WILL FOCUS ON TODAY

_____

_____

_____

_____

MY PRAYER

_____

_____

_____

_____

DAY 4

Scripture: **HOSEA 2:19–20**

I will make you my wife forever, showing you righteousness and justice, unfailing love and compassion. I will be faithful to you and make you mine, and you will finally know me as the LORD.

DEVOTIONAL THOUGHT

God used the prophet Hosea to point out the pain of infidelity. Israel was unfaithful to her husband, the Lord Almighty. But there was good news: God was merciful. His love never failed.

Our society has a way of dealing with failure. We crucify people in the press with facts and innuendos. When we fail, we can accept society's assessment or we can accept God's assessment, which usually relates to His unchanging characteristics. ("I will be faithful to you"; "I will show you righteousness and justice"). What message will you hang on to today?

TRUTH I WILL FOCUS ON TODAY

_____

_____

_____

_____

MY PRAYER

_____

_____

_____

_____

DAY 5

Scripture: ISAIAH 41:10

Don't be afraid, for I am with you. Don't be discouraged, for I am your God. I will strengthen you and help you. I will hold you up with my victorious right hand.

DEVOTIONAL THOUGHT

Ever wish you had a bodyguard or some other strong advocate? The times when we mess up are the times when we most need someone to take our side and remind us that we're not totally worthless. According to the prophet Isaiah, God promises to be that strong advocate. Consider the fact that this assurance is part of the promise to restore Israel after a future period of exile. In other words, God knew they would blow it and He had a plan in place to restore them.

In need of a rescue? The Lord promises to "strengthen you and help you."

TRUTH I WILL FOCUS ON TODAY

_____

_____

_____

_____

MY PRAYER

_____

_____

_____

_____

DAY 6

Scripture: ISAIAH 40:29–31

He gives power to the weak and strength to the powerless. Even youths will become weak and tired, and young men will fall in exhaustion. But those who trust in the LORD will find new strength. They will soar high on wings like eagles. They will run and not grow weary. They will walk and not faint.

DEVOTIONAL THOUGHT

The image of the eagle coasting on an updraft is a powerful one. Imagine soaring like an eagle or living in an aerie on a high cliff. For many of us, though, the image of a small bird frantically beating its wings against a gale-force wind is about all we can come up with.

Some of life's problems leave us powerless and empty—a mere husk. Consider God's promise of renewed power. This is the power that causes us to soar. Overwhelmed? What burdens do you need to strip off and hand to the Lord?

TRUTH I WILL FOCUS ON TODAY

_____

_____

_____

_____

MY PRAYER

_____

_____

_____

_____

DAY 7

Scripture: MATTHEW 10:29–31

What is the price of two sparrows—one copper coin? But not a single sparrow can fall to the ground without your Father knowing it. And the very hairs on your head are all numbered. So don't be afraid; you are more valuable to God than a whole flock of sparrows.

DEVOTIONAL THOUGHT

What are you worth? When life takes a turn for the worse, we can feel as if our value has plummeted. We're somehow not worth as much when we fail. Ever feel like that? Think about the fact that God minors in minutiae. As Jesus assured the disciples, God knows the amount of hair on your head (or in your hairbrush). He knows about every detail of your life.

Now think about someone you love: a spouse, a son or daughter, a friend. Think about the worth that person has in your eyes. God's love for you goes beyond even that. Knowing this, what concerns will you bring to Him today?

TRUTH I WILL FOCUS ON TODAY

_____

_____

_____

_____

MY PRAYER

_____

_____

_____

_____

WEEKLY PROGRESS AND GOALS

❖ Current weight: _____

❖ Pounds lost this week: _____

NEW INSIGHTS

❖ About myself:

_____

_____

❖ From Scripture:

_____

_____

❖ About weight loss:

_____

_____

PLAN FOR NEXT WEEK

❖ Personal issue to focus on:

_____

_____

❖ Biblical truth to live out:

_____

_____

❖ Food to eliminate or restrict for the week:

_____

_____

❖ Exercise goals:

_____

_____

INTRODUCTION

School had always come easy for Jessica. She never really had to study that much, even through college. But graduate school was a different story. Prior to grad school, Jessica's teachers and professors always encouraged, challenged, and affirmed her. In grad school, however, she had a professor who was determined to bring her down for some reason.

In order to finish her master's degree, Jessica had to take a comprehensive examination—eight hours of testing. One day, that professor/advisor called Jessica into his office and in no uncertain terms told her he thought she would fail the exam, that she didn't have what was needed. Tears forming in her eyes, Jessica hurried out of the professor's office and toward home. She shared her devastation with a friend and her family. What now? Although she wanted to give up and quit right then, somehow Jessica decided that she was going to prove her professor wrong.

Immediately, Jessica began an intense study routine, at least two hours a day—starting two months before the exam. Eventually she studied more for that exam than she had ever studied in her four years at college. Jessica went into her exam with confidence and passed with ease.

Jessica could have allowed the pain she felt from her professor's remarks to shut her down and cause her to give up, but she chose to let this hurt motivate and push her to make a change—to study harder and pass the exam.

Every person has similar choices to make. Do we allow our pain to keep us from moving forward, or do we allow it to motivate us to change our lifestyles?

VIDEO 15

Notes from video:

_____

_____

_____

_____

_____

_____

_____

LIFL CONCEPT 15

GOD DOES NOT WANT YOU TO LIVE IN GUILT AND SHAME, BUT INSTEAD TO ALLOW THE PAIN YOU HAVE EXPERIENCED TO MOTIVATE YOU TO MAKE CHANGES IN THE WAY YOU LIVE.

You may have heard this statement: *Our challenges can make us bitter or better.* That may seem trite (and it's much easier to say than do), but it's true. As we've discussed in previous sessions, no one is perfect—everyone sins, makes mistakes, and experiences setbacks and letdowns. And we live in a fallen world; that is, we are surrounded by other sinners who also do wrong and mess up. Things break, bad weather blows in, sickness strikes, people disappoint, insects bite, and traffic jams. We live with those painful and often disappointing realities.

But we do have control over how we will respond to our problems and setbacks. We can't choose much of what happens around us or to us, but we *can choose* our attitudes. When confronted with a challenge, we can choose to meet it head on and conquer it. When dealing with pain, we can use it to motivate us to change for the better and move forward. Then we can take what we've learned and minister to someone else.

What challenges do you face? What choices are you making?

SCRIPTURE

MARK 2:1–12

When Jesus returned to Capernaum several days later, the news spread quickly that he was back home. Soon the house where he was staying was so packed with visitors that there was no more room, even outside the door. While he was preaching God's word to them, four men arrived carrying a paralyzed man on a mat. They couldn't bring him to Jesus because of the crowd, so they dug a hole through the roof above his head. Then they lowered the man on his mat, right down in front of Jesus. Seeing their faith, Jesus said to the paralyzed man, "My child, your sins are forgiven."

But some of the teachers of religious law who were sitting there thought to themselves, "What is he saying? This is blasphemy! Only God can forgive sins!"

Jesus knew immediately what they were thinking, so he asked the, "Why do you question this in your hearts? Is it easier to say to the paralyzed man 'Your sins are forgiven,' or 'Stand up, pick up your mat, and walk'? So I will prove to you that the Son of Man has the authority on earth to forgive sins." Then Jesus turned to the paralyzed man and said, "Stand up, pick up your mat, and go home!"

And the man jumped up, grabbed his mat, and walked out through the stunned onlookers. They were all amazed and praised God, exclaiming, "We've never seen anything like this before!"

The last two Concepts have covered a lot of hopeful ground. Our central emotional trigger (hunger for love) has been disarmed, and our expectations of a free and easy life have been adjusted to a more realistic outlook by our clay-like experiences in life. It's time for another up close and personal reality check.

Have these Concepts connected with you or are they still out there where you can see them but not yet reach them? You know God loves you, and you understand you're like a lump of clay sitting on the potter's wheel. But that's it. You're not moving. You're stuck, frozen, paralyzed. What you are most aware of is guilt and shame over what you have done and left undone. You now know a lot more than you did even a few weeks ago, but you can't stop berating yourself for not acting on what you *did know.* Some of the Concepts you've thought about recently seem painfully obvious. You feel foolish not to have done more sooner, and now you suspect that it might even be hypocritical to start applying the LIFL Concepts when you have already missed so many opportunities along the way.

Welcome to the moment of spiritual paralysis. We've been waiting for you. We knew you would get here. And we've got good news for you—Someone's waiting to talk to you about where you are at this moment.

The best way to understand how Jesus addresses our paralysis of guilt and shame is to see how He handled someone else's. The Bible passage for this session does just that, in an almost Keystone Kops routine. After you read the Mark 2:1–12 passage again, take a moment to visualize it in high-speed video.

Four friends are sitting around, with a fifth one who has been paralyzed for a long time. They want to encourage him but have run out of words. Someone runs in with news—Jesus is back in town! Reports have been spreading that He heals sick people. Maybe, just maybe, Jesus can do something for their paralyzed friend. The four hold a quick huddle in the corner. Before their friend on the mat can object, his friends hoist him like a body toss at a rock concert, and double-time it toward the house where Jesus is staying.

About a block away, they see trouble—the house is packed. So is the area in front of the house and all the windows. What can they do? Then one of the friends, a builder, remembers how the roof of this particular house has been constructed. He knows the interior layout. He calls for another quick huddle. The mat-man begins to wonder what's going to happen. They hoist him again and climb quickly up the stairway on the outside of the house that leads to the rooftop porch. Soon his friends are peeling back the mud and thatch from the center of the roof, making a long opening between the rafters. One of them fastens ropes to each corner of the mat and then the maiden voyage of the original elevator begins.

The roof rubble dropping into the house has created both curiosity and an open spot in front of Jesus. The lowered mat ends up on the floor at His feet. The friends have presented mat-man and his obvious problem to the One they believe can help him. Jesus looks down and speaks, not to the obvious problem but to the deeper one: "My child, your sins are forgiven" (verse 5). No one understands—except mat-man. He knows what Jesus is talking about. When everyone else begins to argue about Jesus' right to forgive sins and wonders about why Jesus hasn't healed the man, mat-man lays quietly contemplating his forgiveness. If nothing else happens that evening, that paralyzed man will be eternally grateful for his friends' help. And that's when Jesus looks down with a smile and almost as an afterthought commands: "Stand up, pick up your mat, and go home!"

For the sake of this lesson, let's call mat-man's four friends Concept One, Concept Two, Concept Three, and Concept Four. Those first four Concepts came into your life like caring and carrying friends. And by the time you reached Concept Four, you knew that healing and wholeness would involve sacrifice and a different way of living. During Concepts Five through Fourteen, you have probably thought or whispered the favorite word of the spiritually paralyzed: *But.* "But what about this?" or "But what about that?" A thousand paralyzing issues have crowded your mind. You know you've heard a lot of good and hopeful news. Yet the "buts" in your mind have kept the paralysis in place.

Now you are lying helpless at Jesus' feet. You are aware suddenly that the underlying theme in all of LIFL is not what you know but *whom* you know and what you allow Him to do in and through your life. Hear Jesus speak the words of Concept Fifteen into your being: "I do not want you to live in guilt and shame but, instead, to allow the pain you have experienced to motivate you to make changes in the way you live." Then receive the same words Jesus said to mat-man, "My child, your sins are forgiven."

You've become so accustomed to all the obvious needs you have for His help that perhaps you've overlooked the deepest need of all. Until you hear His words of forgiveness, you will remain spiritually paralyzed. The most profound change Jesus wants to bring and continue to bring into your life is something no one else can see—His forgiveness of your sins. You don't have to know the mat-man's sins—Jesus did. And He knows your sins and includes them all in His statement. Jesus offers you forgiveness. If you will continually accept it, people will see the other changes He brings about in you. You will "get up and walk" in ways you can hardly imagine!

DISCUSSION QUESTIONS ABOUT SCRIPTURE

❖ What was mat-man's problem? What did his friends decide to do about it?

_____

_____

_____

_____

_____

❖ What did the four men think Jesus would do for their paralyzed friend?

_____

_____

_____

_____

_____

❖ How did they get him to Jesus?

_____

_____

_____

_____

_____

❖ How do you think the crowd may have responded to seeing a man being let down through a hole in the roof? How did Jesus react?

_____

_____

_____

_____

❖ Why were Jesus' words to the man so shocking to the religious leaders?

_____

_____

_____

_____

❖ Why do you think they were more surprised to see the man get up and walk than to see him receive forgiveness?

_____

_____

_____

_____

❖ Which was the greater gift to the paralyzed man? Why?

_____

_____

_____

_____

CASE STUDY

ADRIANA

Adriana never dealt with "no" very well. Her weight history reflected this. She'd always had a problem with weight. She had dieted like a fiend hoping to get Clark's attention in law school, only to be rejected even when she lost the weight. Then she gained the weight right back within a matter of months.

The same thing happened five years after law school. This time the "no" came from the lips of one of the partners in the law firm where she worked. She had been turned down for partner. "You don't show the same drive as the others," the founding partner said. She quickly fell off her diet and gained ten pounds.

"I keep yo-yoing," said Adriana to her friend. Both women tried the same weight-loss program for the third time in five years. "Maybe I just don't have what it takes to stick with a diet program."

YOUR TURN

❖ When Adriana was successful in losing weight, what caused her success?

_____

_____

_____

_____

_____

❖ Why do you think she is unable to stick with a diet to keep the weight off?

_____

_____

_____

_____

❖ How do you think Adriana feels about her "yo-yoing"?

_____

_____

_____

_____

❖ What should she do?

_____

_____

_____

_____

AS A GROUP

❖ What makes some commitments so difficult to keep?

_____

_____

_____

_____

❖ When we fall, fail, or flounder, what choices do we have?

_____

_____

_____

_____

_____

❖ What role can friends play in helping us make the right choice?

_____

_____

_____

_____

_____

❖ How might God use our setbacks and hurts to move us forward, changing our ways and lifestyles?

_____

_____

_____

_____

_____

CHALLENGE

Everyone slips and falls. But not everyone gets up and gets going. Some lie there, feeling guilt and shame; some whine and complain; some blame conditions or others for the situation. While all of those feelings and reactions are understandable, especially in severe conditions and repeated stumbles, there is a better way. Instead of allowing defeats to defeat us (to, in effect, paralyze us), we should use them to strengthen us and motivate us to rise up, try again, and succeed.

This won't be easy. Friends can help bring us—perhaps even carrying us for awhile—to the Savior. The Lord will make all the difference. He will forgive our sins, heal us, and set us on our feet ready to walk and run. But we have a choice.

Will you choose to stay down or get up, to be defeated or victorious?

Daily Devotional Journal

DAY 1

Scripture: 1 CORINTHIANS 6:9–11

Don't you realize that those who do wrong will not inherit the Kingdom of God? Don't fool yourselves. Those who indulge in sexual sin, or who worship idols, or commit adultery, or are male prostitutes, or practice homosexuality, or are thieves, or greedy people, or drunkards, or are abusive, or cheat people—none of these will inherit the Kingdom of God. Some of you were once like that. But you were cleansed; you were made holy; you were made right with God by calling on the name of the Lord Jesus Christ and by the Spirit of our God.

DEVOTIONAL THOUGHT

Ever been a member of an exclusive club? It's a boost for the ego, knowing that you leaped over the hurdle of the membership requirements. Membership in the Kingdom of God is exclusive as well. In fact, this Kingdom is so exclusive, *no one* can meet the membership requirements. One sin will keep you out. Only a sinless Savior can throw the doors open.

Some aspects to our lives we can't change on our own, as Paul's words remind us. We can't change the past or our propensity to err in the same way in the future. Only God can redeem the past and make a future with Him secure. Knowing this does not excuse us from making an effort to live rightly, however. A clean person shouldn't leap back into a mud puddle!

How do your actions show that "you were cleansed; you were made holy"?

TRUTH I WILL FOCUS ON TODAY

_____

_____

_____

_____

MY PRAYER

_____

_____

_____

_____

DAY 2

Scripture: 2 CORINTHIANS 7:9

Now I am glad I sent it, not because it hurt you, but because the pain caused you to repent and change your ways. It was the kind of sorrow God wants his people to have, so you were not harmed by us in any way.

DEVOTIONAL THOUGHT

Being reprimanded is never easy. Under his authority as an apostle, Paul wrote to the believers in and around Corinth, rebuking them as a parent would an erring child. Their repentance in response to his rebuke merited the above debriefing. He commended them for their willingness to change.

There are two ways we can respond to a word of rebuke. We can complain ("This is unfair!") or we can adapt and change. How will you respond to a word of correction?

TRUTH I WILL FOCUS ON TODAY

_____

_____

_____

_____

MY PRAYER

_____

_____

_____

_____

DAY 3

Scripture: JOHN 8:9–11

When the accusers heard this, they slipped away one by one, beginning with the oldest, until only Jesus was left in the middle of the crowd with the woman. Then Jesus stood up again and said to the woman, "Where are your accusers? Didn't even one of them condemn you?" "No, Lord," she said. And Jesus said, "Neither do I. Go and sin no more."

DEVOTIONAL THOUGHT

Instead of condemning a woman caught in the act of adultery, Jesus encouraged change through compassion. Perhaps you haven't had this woman's exact experience, but at one time or another you've probably stood within a circle of accusers. Perhaps you have a stone in hand ready to accuse yourself for an indiscretion. Moving on seems impossible. Does life seem like that now? Jesus has the same words of compassion for you. Do you believe them? "Taste and see that the LORD is good. Oh, the joys of those who take refuge in him!" (Psalm 34:8). Then "go and sin no more."

TRUTH I WILL FOCUS ON TODAY

_____

_____

_____

_____

MY PRAYER

_____

_____

_____

_____

DAY 4

Scripture: JOHN 4:13–18

Jesus replied, "Anyone who drinks this water will soon become thirsty again. But those who drink the water I give will never be thirsty again. It becomes a fresh, bubbling spring within them, giving them eternal life." "Please, sir," the woman said, "give me this water! Then I'll never be thirsty again, and I won't have to come here to get water." "Go and get your husband," Jesus told her. "I don't have a husband," the woman replied. Jesus said, "You're right! You don't have a husband—for you have had five husbands, and you aren't even married to the man you're living with now. You certainly spoke the truth!"

DEVOTIONAL THOUGHT

The fact that Jesus talked to a woman in public was shocking enough from a first-century Jewish male perspective. Added to that was the fact that the woman was a Samaritan with an unsavory past. But Jesus didn't dwell on His reputation or the fact that hers could damage it. He went straight to the heart of the matter: she was spiritually parched; He was the ultimate thirst quencher.

This metaphor was really about the gift of the Holy Spirit and eternal life. This gift can redeem any blighted past or present. The best news is that one who partakes *will never thirst again*. Are you thirsty? Drink fully!

TRUTH I WILL FOCUS ON TODAY

_____

_____

_____

_____

MY PRAYER

_____

_____

_____

_____

DAY 5

Scripture: ROMANS 6:17–18

Thank God! Once you were slaves of sin, but now you wholeheartedly obey this teaching we have given you. Now you are free from your slavery to sin, and you have become slaves to righteous living.

DEVOTIONAL THOUGHT

Slavery is bondage, pure and simple. A slave has no rights, no recourse. A slave has to obey, whether he or she feels like obeying. The recipients of Paul's letter would have understood this implicitly, thanks to the system of slavery established by the Romans.

But slavery to sin is more insidious and demeaning. It leads to death and separation from God. That's why the freedom offered by Jesus' sacrifice is cause for rejoicing. We no longer have to live in shame or defeat. Instead, we trade in this darker kind of slavery for a newer model—slavery to hope, joy, and loving others. What will you do today to show where your allegiance lies?

TRUTH I WILL FOCUS ON TODAY

_____

_____

_____

_____

MY PRAYER

_____

_____

_____

_____

DAY 6

Scripture: TITUS 3:4–7

When God our Savior revealed his kindness and love, he saved us, not because of the righteous things we had done, but because of his mercy. He washed away our sins, giving us a new birth and new life through the Holy Spirit. He generously poured out the Spirit upon us through Jesus Christ our Savior. Because of his grace he declared us righteous and gave us confidence that we will inherit eternal life.

DEVOTIONAL THOUGHT

Has there ever been a time in your life when you thought, *I wish I could start over?* A bad credit report. A bad marriage. A crime. Perhaps the mistakes of the past dogged your steps and bayed like a bloodhound. God's grace makes starting over possible.

But Paul's message to Titus is not simply to show how good we have it but to motivate us to respond in kind toward others. When we couldn't start our lives over, God gave us a completely new life to start. There are so many people mired down and broken by their pasts. They need this reminder of God's mercy and grace. Whom can you tell?

TRUTH I WILL FOCUS ON TODAY

_____

_____

_____

_____

MY PRAYER

_____

_____

_____

_____

DAY 7

Scripture: **REVELATION 21:4**

He will wipe every tear from their eyes, and there will be no more death or sorrow or crying or pain. All these things are gone forever.

DEVOTIONAL THOUGHT

The thought of never crying again, never again feeling sorrow is an attractive one, particularly when life serves up a tragedy. Imagine never again watching a child die or a loved one suffer through a bout of cancer. Imagine never again feeling afraid or worthless. That was the vision given to the apostle John—a vision of incredible hope and victory. Perhaps that's why toward the end of the book he could respond with gusto, "Amen! Come, Lord Jesus!" (22:20)

Here on earth we will experience hard times and hard tears. These times and tears cause us to long for heaven. When you read John's words, what do you long for the most?

TRUTH I WILL FOCUS ON TODAY

_____

_____

_____

_____

MY PRAYER

_____

_____

_____

_____

WEEKLY PROGRESS AND GOALS

❖ Current weight: _____

❖ Pounds lost this week: _____

NEW INSIGHTS

❖ About myself:

_____

_____

❖ From Scripture:

_____

_____

❖ About weight loss:

_____

_____

PLAN FOR NEXT WEEK

❖ Personal issue to focus on:

_____

_____

❖ Biblical truth to live out:

_____

_____

❖ Food to eliminate or restrict for the week:

_____

_____

❖ Exercise goals:

_____

_____

INTRODUCTION

Deciding to buy the sailboat he saw advertised, David walked into the secondhand store. Sitting near the back was a beautiful boat—the mast and sail were intact, the bearings were in perfect condition, and the hull looked new—no holes or dents and with a fresh coat of paint. Why would such a beautiful boat cost so little? David found a worker and asked him this question.

"Well," replied the store clerk, "this boat doesn't have a rudder. But it's no big deal. If you ask me, you're getting an amazing bargain for such a beautiful boat. The missing rudder shouldn't make much of a difference. It's small and insignificant."

David purchased the sailboat and its trailer and quickly drove to the nearest lake. With great anticipation, he launched the boat and jumped in. Soon the wind filled the sails and began to move the vessel forward. David felt great, especially with the breeze flowing through his hair. Then a gust from the east pushed him to the west. It wasn't where he wanted to go but no problem. Soon, however, it became a problem as rocks came into view. Leaning and pulling on the sail, he changed direction a bit, but he still was way off course and far from the launch. That's when he realized the importance of that little rudder.

Little things can make a big difference. Take, for example, our mouths and what we put in them. It may not seem like much, but the discipline (or lack of discipline) that we exercise in this area can affect the other areas of our lives. Not having any control of our eating is similar to how a sailboat reacts without a rudder—no matter how hard we try, without proper steering, we'll just keep heading in the wrong direction.

VIDEO 16

Notes from video:

_____

_____

_____

_____

_____

_____

_____

LIFL CONCEPT 16

WHEN WE CONTROL WHAT WE PUT IN OUR MOUTHS, OTHER AREAS OF OUR LIVES COME UNDER CONTROL ALSO. BUT WHEN OUR EATING IS OUT OF CONTROL, MANY OTHER AREAS WILL NEED TO CHANGE ALONG WITH OUR EATING.

Parents often mention the word *discipline* in discussions about child rearing. Coaches also use this term when describing successful athletic training and game performance. Sometimes we equate discipline with "punishment" as in, "Many parents discipline their children by taking away privileges." But discipline is a positive word implying training and self-control. Although it may involve punishment in certain situations, the goal of discipline is not punitive but progressive, attempting to help that person grow and become "self-disciplined." A disciplined person knows what to do and does it—no procrastination or excuses, no evading responsibility or passing the buck. This person takes responsibility for his or her attitudes, actions, and accomplishments.

Discipline and self-control begin in the small, seemingly insignificant areas—words held back, daily exercise routines, and, yes, our mouth intake. In fact, if we can control our eating—discipline ourselves in that area—we probably will be able to control the other areas of our lives. But the converse is true as well: lack of control in that crucial area probably will lead to problems elsewhere.

So how are you doing with what you put in your mouth? That's where self-control begins.

SCRIPTURE

JAMES 3:1–12

Dear brothers and sisters, not many of you should become teachers in the church, for we who teach will be judged more strictly. Indeed, we all make many mistakes. For if we could control our tongues, we would be perfect and could also control ourselves in every other way.

We can make a large horse go wherever we want by means of a small bit in its mouth. And a small rudder makes a huge ship turn wherever the pilot chooses to go, even though the winds are strong. In the same way, the tongue is a small thing that makes grand speeches.

But a tiny spark can set a great forest on fire. And the tongue is a flame of fire.

It is a whole world of wickedness, corrupting your entire body. It can set your whole life on fire, for it is set on fire by hell itself.

People can tame all kinds of animals, birds, reptiles, and fish, but no one can tame the tongue. It is restless and evil, full of deadly poison. Sometimes it praises our Lord and Father, and sometimes it curses those who have been made in the image of God. And so blessing and cursing come pouring out of the same mouth. Surely, my brothers and sisters, this is not right! Does a spring of water bubble out with both fresh water and bitter water? Does a fig tree produce olives, or a grapevine produce figs? No, and you can't draw fresh water from a salty spring.

The mouth may be the busiest two-way intersection in a person's life. The inbound lane carries life-sustaining food and drink, while the outbound lane carries much of our communication with the outside world. What goes in and out of our mouths has a definite impact on everything else about us. Our sense of self-control hinges on our ability to control our mouths. This importance is highlighted on the intake side by Concept Sixteen. James 3 focuses on the output side.

James wasn't proclaiming a new revelation to his readers. He used what they already understood about horses, ships, and fires to help them recognize the inordinate power of the tongue. What we say can give us a ride or throw us, steer us or sink us, warm us or send our lives up in flames. These vivid pictures of the life-giving or lethal potential in our tongues provide us with sober warnings.

Another ancient example also applies to the *eating* role of our mouths. The people in James's day protected themselves in cities surrounded by massive walls. Many of those walls still stand, thousands of years after the cities have ceased to exist. But even a massive wall couldn't keep a city alive if it had no gates. The city gates were necessary weak points in the otherwise impregnable walls. Gates, like bits, rudders, and sparks represent control points. The main gate was the mouth of a city. As long as the gate was under control, the city was under control.

James could tell his readers, "If we could control our tongues, we would be perfect and could also control ourselves in every other way" (James 3:2). His statement closely parallels Concept Sixteen: "When we control what we put in our mouths, other areas of our lives come under control also. But when eating is out of control many other areas need change along with our eating." The traffic may flow in opposite directions, but the subject is control. By applying the LIFL Concepts we are progressively taking control of a specific area of our lives as part of a larger, life-long plan to develop Christlikeness in every area. We are learning to guard the gate.

The fact that we have identified a specific, crucial area of concern means we've isolated a goal; it doesn't mean that meeting that goal is going to be easy. That's why LIFL has to be a long term, lifestyle choice, not a short-term project.

When we monitor the traffic moving in and out of our "gate," we soon note that James was right. What exits out of the gate is clearly more dangerous than what enters. We have Jesus' word on that: "Can't you see that the food you put into your body cannot defile you? Food doesn't go into your heart, but only passes through the stomach and then goes into the sewer." (By saying this, he declared that every kind of food is acceptable in God's eyes.) And then He added, "It is what comes from inside that defiles you. For from within, out of a person's heart, come evil thoughts, sexual immorality, theft, murder, adultery, greed, wickedness, deceit, lustful desires, envy, slander, pride, and foolishness. All these vile things come from within; they are what defile you" (Mark 7:18b–23).

Getting serious about taking control of what we put in our mouths makes even more sense when we see it as part of the big picture. As difficult as this might be, it pales before other challenges. But it can be a healthy and good place to start.

The evidences of lack of control of your appetites may have provided the motivation for becoming involved in LIFL. Several of the Concepts have already addressed the crucial point that our eating habits are simply one of the indicators of deeper issues. The specific guidance about diet and the reordering of eating habits are practical ways you are learning to engage this area. But be prepared for the balance shift effect that will almost always develop any time we focus on change. As you take control of your mouth, other areas in your life where control is lacking will become more evident. Perhaps you will discover that even though you weren't doing much to deal with the problem of food consumption, you were actually consumed with worries, guilt, and thoughts about food and how it was affecting you. Applying LIFL means you are taking specific action and using your time and energy more efficiently. Now you have time to pay attention to other things that have been hiding behind food and weight issues. These can be huge! That's why Concept Seventeen follows Concept Sixteen. You will need help.

In the meantime, realize that you are making progress (despite setbacks) where once you only felt defeated. You are accepting the fact that you have lived your way into the place where you are, and now you are trusting God to help you live your way to a different place that is healthier and marked by contentment. Your "city" is under extensive renovation. You are establishing control over the gate by limiting access. Certain visitors are no longer welcome through your mouth-gate. Others have been informed that they will have only limited access. And you are welcoming new guests who can make a healthy contribution to the city. Above the gate of your life you can post an imaginary sign to which you can refer any time that something unwelcome demands entrance. On that sign you have painted the words: "Under New Management."

Inside the gate, things may look chaotic. You are painfully aware that much more remains to be repaired and rebuilt. But you've made a good start. And Concept Seventeen will help you keep going!

DISCUSSION QUESTIONS ABOUT SCRIPTURE

❖ What word pictures does James use to describe the importance of the tongue?

_____

_____

_____

_____

_____

_____

❖ Why is the mouth so important to the body?

_____

_____

_____

_____

_____

_____

❖ In what ways is the mouth like the main gate in an ancient city's wall?

_____

_____

_____

_____

_____

_____

❖ Why is the mouth, specifically what we put into it, so difficult to control?

_____

_____

_____

_____

_____

❖ How does the way a person controls his or her mouth affect that person's discipline in other areas of life?

_____

_____

_____

_____

❖ What can people learn about themselves by analyzing how they control their mouths?

_____

_____

_____

_____

_____

CASE STUDY

CANDACE

Candace, like others in her family, always struggled with her weight and self-esteem. Fearful thoughts like *I'm going to be fat* preyed on her mind. She also struggled with guilt over a past drug addiction.

After she became pregnant with her son and was ordered on strict bed rest because of complications, the guilt over her past and her burgeoning weight caused her to eat uncontrollably. Little by little, she gained 100 pounds. Because of her low self-esteem, her marriage suffered as she withdrew from her husband. Even after she gave birth, her eating habits continued. She felt trapped and miserable.

YOUR TURN

❖ What is Candace's struggle?

_____

_____

_____

_____

_____

❖ Why does Candace have a weight problem?

_____

_____

_____

_____

_____

_____

❖ How has this become a vicious cycle for her?

_____

_____

_____

_____

_____

_____

❖ What would you advise Candice to do?

_____

_____

_____

_____

_____

_____

AS A GROUP

❖ Who is the "gatekeeper" of your "wall"? Who should be?

_____

_____

_____

_____

_____

_____

❖ What steps can people take to control what goes in their mouths? Why is this important?

_____

_____

_____

_____

_____

_____

_____

_____

❖ What factors or barriers keep you from guarding the input and output of your mouth?

_____

_____

_____

_____

_____

_____

_____

_____

CHALLENGE

The mouth is a small but vital part of human anatomy. We use it to communicate, to express love and other emotions, and to eat. For being so small, it sure does exert a lot of influence—over ourselves and others.

The discipline needed to Lose It for Life begins right there, at the entrance, the gate. If we can monitor and control what enters there, we usually can control every other area of life. Conversely, lack of discipline in our eating habits will lead to an undisciplined life.

Begin at the beginning, at the gate. Ask God to give you the will and power to watch what you eat. And find a friend to hold you accountable.

DAILY DEVOTIONAL JOURNAL

DAY 1

Scripture: ROMANS 6:12–13

Do not let sin control the way you live; do not give in to sinful desires. Do not let any part of your body become an instrument of evil to serve sin. Instead, give yourselves completely to God, for you were dead, but now you have new life. So use your whole body as an instrument to do what is right for the glory of God.

DEVOTIONAL THOUGHT

Sin is like a rudderless ship heading toward disastrous shoals. That's why Paul urges his readers to take a no tolerance attitude toward it. To stay the course, we would be wise to turn our ship's helm over to God, who is a much more experienced captain.

Once we realize that we've been rescued, we can become a compass of peace for others to follow. We can steer them toward the only rudder guaranteed never to lead them off course. Who do you know right now whose life seems rudderless? What can you do to encourage him or her?

TRUTH I WILL FOCUS ON TODAY

_____

_____

_____

_____

MY PRAYER

_____

_____

_____

_____

DAY 2

Scripture: **1 THESSALONIANS 4:4**

Then each of you will control his own body and live in holiness and honor.

DEVOTIONAL THOUGHT

If you've ever felt out of control (and who hasn't?), Paul's words to the Christians of Thessalonica offer a wellspring of encouragement. In our human experience, our bodily urges (the desire to overeat and other harmful patterns) may seem as controllable as a car without brakes. We feel powerless to change, especially if we've lost control in the past. But holiness reattaches the brake line of our lives, enabling us to steer and avoid a collision.

Think about what being in control and living in holiness and honor might mean. Even if you *can't* imagine this type of life, it *is* possible with the Holy Spirit. As Paul says in 1 Thessalonians 4:3, "God's will is for you to be holy." What God wills for a person to do, He also equips. As the writer of Hebrews explained, "May he equip you with all you need for doing his will. May he produce in you, through the power of Jesus Christ, every good thing that is pleasing to him" (Hebrews 13:21).

What changes do you sense on the horizon as a result of living "in holiness and honor"?

TRUTH I WILL FOCUS ON TODAY

_____

_____

_____

_____

MY PRAYER

_____

_____

_____

_____

DAY 3

Scripture: JEREMIAH 15:19

This is how the LORD responds: "If you return to me, I will restore you so you can continue to serve me. If you speak good words rather than worthless ones, you will be my spokesman. You must influence them; do not let them influence you!"

DEVOTIONAL THOUGHT

Many people think that being "called by God" insulates one from feelings of failure or grief. The prophet Jeremiah would disagree. He grieved over his tough ministry to an unrepentant people. His despair resulted in a rebuke from the Lord and a challenge to Jeremiah to let go of thoughts unworthy of the prophet.

We may read such a passage and shudder at the thought of being rebuked for self-pity. After all, aren't we entitled to feel a little sorry for ourselves when the going gets tough? "No!" says the Lord. As with the prophet Jeremiah, an unbelieving world watches the movements of believers. They form their views of God based on our actions. What message does your behavior proclaim?

TRUTH I WILL FOCUS ON TODAY

_____

_____

_____

_____

MY PRAYER

_____

_____

_____

_____

DAY 4

Scripture: PHILIPPIANS 4:8

And now, dear brothers and sisters, one final thing. Fix your thoughts on what is true, and honorable, and right, and pure, and lovely, and admirable. Think about things that are excellent and worthy of praise.

DEVOTIONAL THOUGHT

Imagine driving a car and not looking at the road ahead but, instead, looking at a person or an object on the side of the road. Fixating on that person or object instead of on what's ahead would probably cause you to crash.

In the same way, we can fix our thoughts on hard words spoken to us, painful experiences of the past, or even lies. These words, experiences, and lies cause us to crash as well. Paul, in his most joy-filled letter, offers a more positive target to fixate upon. You've heard the phrase, "You are what you eat." In other words, what you digest is what you become. If we digest a constant diet of lies, rumors, and despairing statements, our lives will reflect defeat. If we digest that which is true, beautiful, and admirable, our lives will reflect those things as well.

Think of how your senses light up when you see a beautiful sunset, a child's smile, or hear someone affirm you. "Fix your thoughts on what is true."

TRUTH I WILL FOCUS ON TODAY

_____

_____

_____

_____

MY PRAYER

_____

_____

_____

_____

DAY 5

Scripture: **PROVERBS 25:28**

A person without self-control is like a city with broken-down walls.

DEVOTIONAL THOUGHT

A city wall was a necessary protective measure against invading armies. This is why Nehemiah was grieved when he discovered the Jewish exiles had returned to a city with a broken wall (see Nehemiah 1:3–4). Invaders could come and have a field day. In the same way, self-control is a wall protecting our hearts. It keeps enemies such as overeating and destructive sexual habits at bay. But often we feel like the person described in this verse—sorely lacking in self-control.

Self-control isn't like cruise control—a button you push to coast. It still requires an effort of the will. Even a wall needs a watchman to stand guard and warn of enemies who threaten to breach the wall.

What enemies threaten to breach your control? Have you prayed about them?

TRUTH I WILL FOCUS ON TODAY

_____

_____

_____

_____

MY PRAYER

_____

_____

_____

_____

DAY 6

Scripture: GALATIANS 5:22–23

But the Holy Spirit produces this kind of fruit in our lives: love, joy, peace, patience, kindness, goodness, faithfulness, gentleness, and self-control. There is no law against these things!

DEVOTIONAL THOUGHT

If you're a gardener, you know the work that goes into producing a healthy crop—whether flowers, fruit, or vegetables. You're constantly in the soil, weeding, watering, and ultimately waiting for that plant to grow.

Many times, we read Paul's words in Galatians 5 and think that *we* are in the position of gardener. We strain to produce patience or joy or self-control. But as Paul reminds us, the *Holy Spirit* is the gardener who "produces this kind of fruit in our lives." Our job is to keep connected to Him. Are you?

TRUTH I WILL FOCUS ON TODAY

_____

_____

_____

_____

MY PRAYER

_____

_____

_____

_____

DAY 7

Scripture: LUKE 12:29–30

Don't be concerned about what to eat and what to drink. Don't worry about such things. These things dominate the thoughts of unbelievers all over the world, but your Father already knows your needs.

DEVOTIONAL THOUGHT

Jesus was a master at revolutionary thinking. So His advice to avoid worrying about food must have come as a shock to people of an agrarian society, many of whom struggled with hunger and poverty. Today we might say, "You've gotta be kidding, Jesus! I'm always thinking about my next meal," as we consider how hungry we are, thanks to whatever diet we're on. But Jesus' words, as recorded by Luke, are a reminder of life beyond the physical or beyond immediate gratification.

What thoughts dominate your mind these days? Consider Jesus' words. "Your Father already knows your needs."

TRUTH I WILL FOCUS ON TODAY

_____

_____

_____

_____

MY PRAYER

_____

_____

_____

_____

WEEKLY PROGRESS AND GOALS

- ❖ Current weight: _____
- ❖ Pounds lost this week: _____

NEW INSIGHTS

- ❖ About myself:

_____

_____

- ❖ From Scripture:

_____

_____

- ❖ About weight loss:

_____

_____

PLAN FOR NEXT WEEK

- ❖ Personal issue to focus on:

_____

_____

- ❖ Biblical truth to live out:

_____

_____

- ❖ Food to eliminate or restrict for the week:

_____

_____

- ❖ Exercise goals:

_____

_____

INTRODUCTION

With football season about to kick off, Marc decides to buy a new HDTV, plasma, 50-inch flat-screen television. He purchases the equipment, including surround-sound speakers, and then hurries home. With great care, Marc puts everything in place, meticulously attaching the speakers, digital box, control switch, and TV. Eagerly grabbing the remote, he hits "on." Nothing happens. Marc checks the connections and tries again. Nothing. He shakes the remote and then tries hitting the button on the set itself. Still nothing. For an anxious hour, Marc continues to check and recheck every connection. Finally, in desperation, he flips through the yellow pages and calls a TV repair shop. Marc knows the technician will charge fifty bucks just for walking through the door, but it's worth it, he thinks.

The tech arrives, does a quick survey of the unit, walks to the wall, pulls out the power cord from behind the set, and plugs it into the wall. Problem solved in thirty seconds.

Most people have done something like that, sometimes in the most unlikely places or circumstances. Consider weight loss, for example. We can try all the new diets and have the best motivations, but they won't help a bit without the power to turn them on and carry them out. Unless we are plugged into the power Source, we will never meet our goals.

The fact is, we can't change on our own. We need help; we need the power of God to strengthen and energize us.

VIDEO 17

Notes from video:

_____

_____

_____

_____

_____

_____

LIFL CONCEPT 17

THE REASON YOUR EATING PROBLEM STARTED HAS LITTLE TO DO WITH WHY YOU REMAIN LOCKED INTO IT. WHEN YOU SURRENDER TO GOD, HE GIVES YOU EVERY-THING YOU NEED TO CHANGE.

Nothing is more frustrating than to experience what Marc did—to be unplugged, oblivious to the power at his fingertips. Not all of life's challenges can be solved so simply, but the principle is clear: all the plans, techniques, programs, and accessories won't work without the *power*.

Today's concept is all about power, God's power. He has everything we need to change, and He promises to give it to us if we will just permit Him to do so. This means surrendering to Him—giving in, yielding to His control.

Thinking, planning, strategizing, and, even, working hard are important. But the power to keep going and to change for life comes from God. Plug in!

SCRIPTURE

2 TIMOTHY 1:7–14

For God has not given us a spirit of fear and timidity, but of power, love, and self-discipline.

So never be ashamed to tell others about out Lord. And don't be ashamed of me, either, even though I'm in prison for him. With the strength God gives you, be ready to suffer with me for the sake of the Good News. For God saved us and called us to live a holy life. He did this, not because we deserved it, but because that was his plan from before the beginning of time—to show us his grace through Christ Jesus. And now he has made all of this plain to us by the appearing of Christ Jesus, our Savior. He broke the power of death and illuminated the way to life and immortality through the Good News. And God chose me to be a preacher, an apostle, and a teacher of this Good News.

That is why I am suffering here in prison. But I am not ashamed of it, for I know the one I whom I trust, and I am sure that he is able to guard what I have entrusted to him until the day of his return.

Hold on to the pattern of wholesome teaching you learned from me—a pattern shaped by the faith and love that you have in Christ Jesus. Through the power of

the Holy Spirit who lives within us, carefully guard the precious truth that has been entrusted to you.

Most of us have had experience with failure. Struggling with our appetites for a long time, we've had repeated setbacks. We have received help from the insight in Concept Six that has equipped us to have a "training" rather than "trying" approach to our problems. We know that "trying" leads to failure and "training" includes and overcomes failure. But we have history. Every time we fall, our past rears up to proclaim our total failure. That's why the realization that we are "cracked pots" (see Concept Fourteen) can be both a humorous and helpful response to failures. We're not going to keep living the way we've always lived.

We need built-in responses to answer the long established patterns in our lives. These patterns have become automatic ways of living, even though we realize they didn't lead to a life we wanted. So we have taken our life-vehicle into the LIFL shop and replaced the transmission with a standard one. We're learning to use a clutch and shift through life. We're paying more attention to how we get where we're going. We're taking driving lessons from the One who designed our vehicle and knows everything about it. We know we've got a long journey ahead.

God does not define us by our failures; He defines us by His love. No, He doesn't ignore our sins and failures. But He's done something about them by covering them with Jesus' sacrifice. Now He doesn't have to deal with us as we deserve. He deals with us out of His love for us.

By all accounts, Timothy was not obvious leadership material. He was probably fairly shy and reluctant to stand in the spotlight and pressure of leadership. He experienced some failures along the way. Where the young man may have felt hopelessness, Paul saw potential, and he gave Timothy assignments that stretched and challenged the young man. But Paul didn't just shove Timothy into the pool and walk away. He spent time with Timothy in the pool, showing by example and instruction how to swim. And when he did push Timothy in the pool, he stood close by, shouting encouragement. The passage for this lesson is one of the shouts to Timothy as he struggled to stay afloat.

In the verses that precede our passage, Paul reminded Timothy of his heritage. He had built-in resources that he could depend on. Timothy had learned from his family and from Paul. The old apostle assured the young pastor that people were pulling for him to do his best. They knew he could swim!

Then, in verse 7, Paul voices his crucial point: We can face whatever we have to face in the present because "God has not given us a spirit of fear and timidity, but of power, love, and self-discipline." This is the message we need to hear when we apply Concept Sixteen and begin to control the mouth-gateway to our lives. Other issues (bigger ones) are going to demand attention and seem impossible to overcome. Our natural inclination may be to react with fear and timidity. The issues we knew about were daunting enough—what next? Concept Seventeen puts things in perspective: "The reason your eating problem started has little to do with why you remain locked into it. When you surrender to God, He gives you everything you need to change."

Our natural "spirit" is characterized by fear and timidity. God replaces it with His Holy Spirit. In one sense, learning to *fear* (reverence) God the right way means that nothing else can frighten us! If God is standing behind us, absolutely nothing can come at us that won't be more afraid of God than we are of it! If the most awesome and fearful Being in the universe and beyond loves us and has our best interest in mind, why would we need to fear anything or anyone else?

Our tendency toward timidity involves a settled lack of confidence when it comes to things that seem impossible. Most of the problems we struggle with in life get that label along the way. Weight control? Impossible! Eating discipline? Impossible! Good spiritual habits? Impossible! Contentment? Really impossible! What we need to remember is that we gave them that label—we call our problems impossible. God doesn't look at them that way. When asked about one of life's "impossibilities," Jesus said, "What is impossible for people is possible for God" (Luke 18:27). One of the most empowering experiences we can have in life is to identify the things we have previously labeled "impossible" and deliberately cover those labels with new ones that read: "With Christ—possible!" Now that's an anti-timidity exercise.

But Paul has a lot more in mind than just re-labeling things. He tells Timothy (and us) that the Holy Spirit makes "power, love, and self-discipline" available to us. God's supply is never exhausted and He is available 24/7. Things we have now labeled "With Christ—possible," we need to prepare new labels for that read, "With Christ—done!" Our understanding of God's power must include the conclusion that if God does not want something in our lives or does want something in our lives, it will be. The issue of "when" will replace the timidity of "if." Confidence in God's will becomes a description of the way we pursue life—"Your will be done today, Lord."

Every time we see a reference to God's love in Scripture, the words of Ephesians 3:16–21 (See Concept Thirteen) ought to fill our minds. "Love" is such a small word—God's love immediately makes it something immeasurable! Why would God help us overcome what looks impossible? Because He loves us. If we need more reasons than that, we need a bigger picture of God's love.

Have you ever thought of self-discipline as a gift? If Someone has made power and love abundantly available to you, wouldn't one of the spin-offs be self-discipline? Is self-discipline something you know you need? Is self-discipline something God desires for you? Then it can't be labeled "impossible." It should be labeled, "With Christ—done."

Paul asked Timothy to take on some difficult challenges. The challenges you face in applying the LIFL principles in daily living are daunting. With everything we are learning about life, we know that at rare times we will be able to confidently say, "It's all under control." But no matter what we face or how often we have faced it in the past, we now have the freedom to joyfully scribble a sticky note saying "With Christ—possible!"and smack it on every problem we face.

DISCUSSION QUESTIONS ABOUT SCRIPTURE

❖ What was Paul's relationship to Timothy?

_____

_____

_____

_____

_____

❖ In this passage, what is Paul's main message to this young man?

_____

_____

_____

_____

_____

❖ What leads to timidity or lack of confidence in general? How about with weight control?

_____

_____

_____

_____

_____

❖ What makes us believe that certain problems are "impossible" to solve?

_____

_____

_____

_____

❖ How can we be confident that with Christ they can be labeled "possible" and, even, "done"?

_____

_____

_____

_____

❖ What can we do to access God's power in our lives?

_____

_____

_____

_____

❖ How can this help us Lose It for Life?

_____

_____

_____

_____

CASE STUDY

RYAN

"Dude! You gotta check out the trainer on staff at the health club."

"I don't need him," Ryan said to his friend Eric, as they walked toward the health club's elliptical machines.

"Seriously, man, he programmed a regimen for me. It's really been more effective than what I was doing on my own. And haven't you been complaining that you haven't taken off the pounds like you want to?"

Ryan shrugged. There was no way he was going to ask the advice of a personal trainer. He didn't feel like hearing what he was doing wrong. He had been a member of this health club for a year now. He saw the same people each week. Some had commented on his diligence. One guy even said he was coming to the health club more regularly because of Ryan's example. Wouldn't consulting a personal trainer make it seem as if he didn't know what he was doing?

Ryan rubbed his sore shoulder. He must have pulled it while on the machine the last time. Oh well. He'd have to tough it out.

YOUR TURN

❖ Why does Ryan come to the health club?

_____

_____

_____

_____

_____

_____

❖ Why does Eric think Ryan needs the help of a trainer?

_____

_____

_____

_____

_____

❖ What keeps Ryan from asking for help?

_____

_____

_____

_____

_____

❖ What do you think will happen with Ryan's fitness and weight loss program?

_____

_____

_____

_____

_____

AS A GROUP

❖ What life patterns tend to keep us from plugging into God's power?

_____

_____

_____

_____

❖ How successful will we be trying to succeed totally on our own?

_____

_____

_____

_____

❖ In what ways will God's power help us succeed?

_____

_____

_____

_____

❖ How can we plug into Him?

_____

_____

_____

_____

CHALLENGE

Many factors keep people from accessing the power available to them. They may have behavior patterns that provide a sense of security—it's the way they've always done it. They may be skeptical, thinking that not even God can help. Or they may simply be too proud to ask for help.

But why not use the power available? God loves us, wants the best for us, and provides amazing resources at our disposal. And, quite frankly, we won't succeed over the long haul without Him. Plug in and power up!

DAILY DEVOTIONAL JOURNAL

DAY 1

Scripture: EZEKIEL 36:26

And I will give you a new heart, and I will put a new spirit in you. I will take out your stony, stubborn heart and give you a tender, responsive heart.

DEVOTIONAL THOUGHT

Here, the prophet Ezekiel continues the prophecy of Israel's coming restoration. One day the nation would no longer stubbornly cling to old ways of behavior, he said. The people's hearts would be transformed from the inside out.

Like the engine of a car, the heart is one of the control centers of the body. We talk of the brain—the neurological impulses to act, and so forth—but the heart is really the center of our desires and attitudes. Imagine having a heart that's pliable instead of rebellious. That's what God promises. But He won't force us to take it. As with any heart transplant, the old one has to be taken out of the body and replaced with the new one.

What does having "a new spirit" and "a tender, responsive heart" mean to you?

TRUTH I WILL FOCUS ON TODAY

_____

_____

_____

_____

MY PRAYER

_____

_____

_____

_____

DAY 2

Scripture: MATTHEW 10:38–39

If you refuse to take up your cross and follow me, you are not worthy of being mine. If you cling to your life, you will lose it; but if you give up your life for me, you will find it.

DEVOTIONAL THOUGHT

Picture a yellow or red leaf clinging tenaciously to a tree in a fall breeze. Seems ludicrous, doesn't it, considering that (a) the leaf is technically dead, and (b) eventually the wind will pull it off the branch. But we're sometimes like that leaf. We think we can cling to our lives—our agendas—and follow Christ. But as Jesus explained in no uncertain terms, we can't hang on to both. Technically, we're supposed to be "dead" to ourselves, "since we have died to sin," Paul proclaims in Romans 6:2. So what are we hanging on to?

TRUTH I WILL FOCUS ON TODAY

_____

_____

_____

_____

MY PRAYER

_____

_____

_____

_____

DAY 3

Scripture: ROMANS 6:6–7

We know that our old sinful selves were crucified with Christ so that sin might lose its power in our lives. We are no longer slaves to sin. For when we died with Christ we were set free from the power of sin.

DEVOTIONAL THOUGHT

Sometimes when you're having trouble with a computer, you have to shut it down in order to get the power to cycle through it correctly. That way, the glitches that affected its performance might disappear.

As Christians, we have to power down and die to ourselves completely, "so that sin might lose its power in our lives." The old attitudes that cycle through us can no longer be rebooted. At least that's the plan. But sometimes we plug back into the old pattern of thinking and behaving. We forget that we're set free!

What do you need to "disconnect" from today as a reminder of your freedom through Christ?

TRUTH I WILL FOCUS ON TODAY

_____

_____

_____

_____

MY PRAYER

_____

_____

_____

_____

DAY 4

Scripture: JOHN 17:11

Now I am departing from the world; they are staying in this world, but I am coming to you. Holy Father, you have given me your name; now protect them by the power of your name so that they will be united just as we are.

DEVOTIONAL THOUGHT

Jesus' prayer for His disciples shows the power and unity available to us through the Holy Spirit. We're absolutely powerless without the Holy Spirit. Unity is nonexistent without a union with the triune God, who unites and protects us "by the power of [His] name." We all crave power. Yet, we have no power on our own. As spiritual sheep we easily fall prey to any wolf on the prowl. And wolves are good at separating a flock—sending the weak and helpless off on their own. Easy pickings.

Perhaps you feel alone in your struggle to change your life. Maybe you feel cornered by various "wolves"—fear, frustration, disappointment. You're not alone and defenseless. By the name of Jesus, you have the power—His power.

TRUTH I WILL FOCUS ON TODAY

_____

_____

_____

_____

MY PRAYER

_____

_____

_____

_____

DAY 5

Scripture: HEBREWS 1:3

The Son radiates God's own glory and expresses the very character of God, and he sustains everything by the mighty power of his command. When he had cleansed us from our sins, he sat down in the place of honor at the right hand of the majestic God in heaven.

DEVOTIONAL THOUGHT

Just as the moon reflects the sun's light, the Son reflects the light of God—His glory and nature, as the writer of Hebrews declares. Unlike the moon, which can only reflect light rather than produce it, the Son has the same characteristics as the Father. "Anyone who has seen me has seen the Father," Jesus declared (John 14:9). Therefore, Christ has the authority to cleanse us from our propensity to sin. Cleansed and forgiven, we too reflect His glory and character. What are some ways you can radiate God's light to others?

TRUTH I WILL FOCUS ON TODAY

_____

_____

_____

_____

MY PRAYER

_____

_____

_____

_____

DAY 6

Scripture: 2 CORINTHIANS 13:4

Although he was crucified in weakness, he now lives by the power of God. We, too, are weak, just as Christ was, but when we deal with you we will be alive with him and will have God's power.

DEVOTIONAL THOUGHT

In answer to the questions and debates of the believers of Corinth, debates sparked by false teachers who seemed to have it all together, Paul once again repeated the gospel message: Jesus died and rose again. He didn't come as a powerful Messiah, ready to smite His enemies. He came to die the death of a common criminal.

Jesus' example of meekness is sometimes misinterpreted as weakness or lacking strength. But true meekness is power under control. Jesus went to the cross because it was God's will and was necessary to pay the price for sin. He could have stopped the atrocity at any time, but He didn't. Now, all authority is His because He chose to submit to the authority of the Father. We also have the power to live in freedom.

TRUTH I WILL FOCUS ON TODAY

_____

_____

_____

_____

MY PRAYER

_____

_____

_____

_____

DAY 7

Scripture: 1 CORINTHIANS 2:3–5

I came to you in weakness—timid and trembling. And my message and my preaching were very plain. Rather than using clever and persuasive speeches, I relied only on the power of the Holy Spirit. I did this so you would trust not in human wisdom but in the power of God.

DEVOTIONAL THOUGHT

Paul chose not to appeal to these Christians through a show of personal prowess but, instead, to rely on the power of the Spirit. Paul's humble example here mirrored Jesus' humility. Although Paul didn't lack the ability to give a good argument—he was a Pharisee after all and well educated (see Philippians 3:5)—he didn't need the applause or affirmation such a gesture would bring.

And that's really the crux of the matter, isn't it? In a society where weakness is despised and strength revered, we fear appearing weak and helpless. But our weakness shows our dependence on God's strength.

TRUTH I WILL FOCUS ON TODAY

_____

_____

_____

_____

MY PRAYER

_____

_____

_____

_____

WEEKLY PROGRESS AND GOALS

❖ Current weight: _____

❖ Pounds lost this week: _____

NEW INSIGHTS

❖ About myself:

_____

_____

❖ From Scripture:

_____

_____

❖ About weight loss:

_____

_____

PLAN FOR NEXT WEEK

❖ Personal issue to focus on:

_____

_____

❖ Biblical truth to live out:

_____

_____

❖ Food to eliminate or restrict for the week:

_____

_____

❖ Exercise goals:

_____

_____

INTRODUCTION

Kids say the funniest things, and sometimes the most embarrassing things. Where in the world do they learn those interesting words and phrases? Usually from the people closest to them—their parents. Someone lightheartedly once said, "Children seldom misquote you. In fact, they usually repeat word for word what you shouldn't have said." Your children are always watching you.

We are examples, for good or bad, to the people in our lives. Children pick up values and habits modeled by their parents. For example, men whose fathers beat them may find themselves hitting their own children. Children from broken homes often repeat that pattern. Boys can learn that "Grown men don't cry." Overweight parents often have overweight children.

The choices we make affect not just ourselves but the people who surround us. And here's something interesting that psychologists have discovered: Adults who believe their children are turning out well feel better about themselves. And the more parents see themselves as the reason for those results, the better the parents feel. It's one big loop.

VIDEO 18

Notes from video:

_____

_____

_____

_____

_____

_____

_____

_____

_____

_____

_____

LIFL CONCEPT 18

MY LIFE IS NOT ALL ABOUT ME; BECAUSE MY CHILDREN AND OTHERS ARE WATCHING ME AND FOLLOWING MY LEAD, I NEED TO BE A GOOD EXAMPLE OF HEALTHY LIVING.

A person doesn't have to win an election, be chosen "captain," own a business, head up an organization, or win a race to be a leader. In his or her own way, every person leads someone. One of the more obvious and vital contexts is family, where the parents lead by example and direction. Children pick up Mom and Dad's values, habits, and ways of reacting to stress and problems. Our neighbors, co-workers, church members, relatives, and friends all learn from our example, for better or for worse. So the question is simply, "What kind of example am I?"

SCRIPTURE

MARK 12:26–34

"But now, as to whether the dead will be raised—haven't you ever read about this in the writings of Moses, in the story of the burning bush? Long after Abraham, Isaac, and Jacob had died, God said to Moses, 'I am the God of Abraham, the God of Isaac, and the God of Jacob.' So he is the God of the living, not the dead. You have made a serious error."

One of the teachers of religious law was standing there listening to the debate. He realized that Jesus had answered well, so he asked, "Of all the commandments, which is the most important?"

Jesus replied, "The most important commandment is this: 'Listen, O Israel! The Lord our God is the one and only Lord. And you must love the Lord your God with all your heart, all your soul, all your mind, and all your strength.' The second is equally important: 'Love your neighbor as yourself.' No other commandment is greater than these."

The teacher of religious law replied, "Well said, Teacher. You have spoken the truth by saying that there is only one God and no other. And I know it is important to love him with all my heart and all my understanding and all my strength, and to love my neighbor as myself. This is more important than to offer all of the burnt offerings and sacrifices required in the law."

Realizing how much the man understood, Jesus said to him, "You are not far from the Kingdom of God." And after that, no one dared to ask him any more questions.

We began a difficult journey back in LIFL Concept One. Taking responsibility for constructing the prisons and forging the chains that hold us captive wasn't an easy first step. But slowly and carefully we have taken more steps to deal with the difficulties created by efforts to get our lives turned around and headed in the right direction.

Seventeen Concepts later, we come to a final, liberating step! The journey that began with a truthful look inward comes to an end with a step outward, into our world. Everything we've learned and thought about impacts us, to be sure, but it also affects those around us. We are ready to declare Concept Eighteen, "My life is not all about me; because my children and others are watching me and following my lead, I need to be a good example of healthy living."

The nature of the LIFL Concepts is that they point to cycles of discovery in life. They are not points we reach that we leave behind forever. Rather, they are stages in a life that cycles upward, taking us through the same lessons over and over at new levels as we apply what we learn. Adopting Concept Eighteen sets the stage for our return to Concept One for a fresh look at self-inflicted limitations in life.

Everyone wants to know the bottom line. We would like to grasp a central idea that's big enough to grab our attention and occupy our efforts in one way or another every day of our lives. That quest brings us to this lesson's Bible passage. It describes a conversation that occurred during Jesus' last week on earth.

Jesus had been hounded all day with trick questions. One little group after another had approached Him with what they thought was a question that would stun and silence Him. To their shock, the effect was reversed and a steady stream of silenced opponents wandered away from Him, dazed. Those who watched were amazed. Jesus' enemies came with tricks, conundrums, and puzzles; He responded with probing questions and truth.

One man in the crowd found himself completely disarmed by Jesus' forthrightness. Perhaps he was part of a group waiting its turn to cross-examine Jesus. But at some point, with admiration ringing in his voice, this teacher of the religious law asked a personal question. We can be eternally grateful, because he asked the one question each of us would eventually pose to Jesus if we were in that man's place, "Of all the commandments, which is the most important?" (Mark 12:28). Maybe we wouldn't use those exact words, but we want to know what it's all about. What's the central truth, the main thing, the most important priority?

We know the tone of this man's question was genuine because Jesus responded in a different way. His other questioners were met with return questions, challenges, and table-turning statements from Jesus. This man got a straight answer. Jesus looked him in the eye and began to speak words that rang with familiarity in that man's soul. Jesus recited

Deuteronomy 6:4–5, the Shema, which was the formal prayer used twice daily by faithful Jews. This man had probably already said these words that day. But Jesus linked the first command to love God with everything we've got with another Old Testament command—to love our neighbor as ourselves (Leviticus 19:18).

Like the eighteen Concepts of LIFL, the Great Commandment begins and ends with what *we* must do. There is an implied "you" in these commands. First, you must love the Lord your God; second, you must love your neighbor; third, you must love yourself. This is not the order of our experience, but it is the order of obedience we should follow.

The order of experience starts before the Great Commandment. In that order, *God acts first* by loving us. We love after and because He first loved us (see 1 John 4:19). Our love at its very best is always responding, never initiating. Changed and inspired by God's love, in turn we respond in love to God, to others, to ourselves. It has often been pointed out that "loving ourselves" in its basic form is raw self-interest more than genuine self-sacrificing love. But even this untamed material serves Jesus' purpose. If we love others with the same raw self-interest that we apply to ourselves, we will seek the best for them. That pursuit will grow into genuine love as we learn the sacrificial and tender parts of the authentic love that God is delighted to teach us in Christ. No doubt about it—life in Christ will be a tenderizing experience! Eventually, the more we experience and learn about God's love, the more we will enjoy simply letting ourselves be embraced by it. The love that we need to carry out the Great Commandment comes generously from God Himself.

The trapped condition that we faced back in Concept One meant, among other things, that we are incapable of loving others the way they ought to be loved, as Jesus demonstrated. As we apply the Concepts, we are loosening bonds that have held us captive for a long time. But one of the proofs of our growing freedom comes as we look up from our chains and beyond our prisons into the lives of others and see their needs in a clear, new, loving way. Our self-made captivity also kept our attention captive. Freedom really means we can genuinely care for others. We discover a whole new level of benefit when life isn't about us any more.

The man who asked the question of Jesus that day agreed profoundly with the answer Jesus gave him. But Jesus wasn't finished with the man. Jesus wanted to give him much more than an answer; Jesus offered him a life. With what must have been an inviting smile, Jesus said, "You are not far from the Kingdom of God" (Mark 12:34). The Gospels don't record the man's response. The man could have responded, "How do I get all the way?" or "Can you take me the rest of the way, Lord?" We don't know. What we *can* know is *our* response.

What is our response to the Eighteen Concepts? What's our response to the open door of freedom that stands before us? What's our response to the needs of those around us who need our love and healthy presence? What will you say to Jesus by your living choices today? Do you know where you are in relation to the Kingdom of God?

Discussion Questions about Scripture

❖ Why did the man ask Jesus the question about the "greatest commandment"?

_____

_____

_____

_____

_____

❖ Why did Jesus take him seriously?

_____

_____

_____

_____

_____

❖ What was Jesus' answer?

_____

_____

_____

_____

_____

❖ What does it mean for us to love God with all of our "heart, soul, mind, and strength"?

_____

_____

_____

_____

❖ What do you think Jesus meant by loving our "neighbor"?

_____

_____

_____

_____

❖ Why is loving others, at times, more difficult than loving God?

_____

_____

_____

_____

_____

_____

❖ How can our experience with LIFL help us fulfill this commandment?

_____

_____

_____

_____

_____

CASE STUDY

JANELLE

"Cara! It's nearly dinnertime!" Janelle called upstairs to her daughter. "Come down."

"I'm not hungry, Mom!" Cara called back, although her voice had a muffled quality.

Instantly suspicious, Janelle walked upstairs and entered her daughter's room in time to see her stuff an Oreo in her mouth. "Cara Elise, didn't I just tell you dinner would be ready soon? And you're eating those? Honestly!"

"Sorry," Cara tried to say over a mouthful of Oreo cookie.

Janelle returned to the kitchen, where her husband, Philip, had just lifted the lid to a pot and dipped a spoon in. He grinned at her as he spooned soup over a slice of buttered bread.

"Honestly, Phil, you should've seen Cara sneaking Oreos." She hastily cut up a carrot to add to a salad. After tossing it into the bowl, she popped a slice in her mouth. "You'd think she didn't notice how we struggled all last year with losing weight. I'd hate for her to have to go through that. That's why I try to make healthy meals." She popped another carrot slice in her mouth.

Philip nodded as he grabbed a few chips out of an open bag on the counter. "Phil!" Janelle said, scandalized. "I just said dinner will be ready soon."

YOUR TURN

❖ Why was Janelle upset with her daughter, Cara?

_____

_____

_____

_____

_____

❖ What's wrong with what Cara was doing?

_____

_____

_____

_____

❖ Where do you think she picked up that habit? Why?

_____

_____

_____

_____

AS A GROUP

❖ Today how would Jesus answer the question, "Who is my neighbor?"

_____

_____

_____

_____

❖ In what ways can the example we help set fulfill Jesus' command to love our neighbors as ourselves?

_____

_____

_____

_____

❖ Who might be watching you and following your example?

_____

_____

_____

_____

_____

_____

❖ If someone were to say, "Losing weight is *my* problem, no one else's," how would you answer him or her?

_____

_____

_____

_____

_____

_____

CHALLENGE

Although the LIFL program is very focused and personal and highlights what we, as individuals, should do for ourselves, its effects can also be far reaching. That's because whether we like it or not, we influence others by what we do and say. We are living examples, positively or negatively. No one lives totally to himself or herself.

This is especially true for moms and dads. Children pick up their parents' values, habits, and lifestyles. Thus, adults with poor eating and exercising routines will produce kids with the same—and usually with the same bad results in weight and health.

When Jesus said the second greatest commandment involves loving others as ourselves, He knew that often the most difficult people to love are those closest to us. Yet that's where love must begin. It's tough because they know us so well—and we know them. Being serious about our commitment to Christ, however, means obeying Him, and that begins at home.

What kind of example are you? What style of personal discipline do people learn from watching how you live? It's not just about you—and it's not just about now.

DAILY DEVOTIONAL JOURNAL

DAY 1

Scripture: 1 JOHN 2:10

Anyone who loves another brother or sister is living in the light and does not cause others to stumble.

DEVOTIONAL THOUGHT

When you walk into a dark room, you turn on a light to avoid stumbling over furniture. When you love a brother or sister, the apostle John explains, you're lighting up the darkness as well as helping a brother or sister avoid stumbling into sin. The contrast between the light and the darkness is one John used throughout this letter to help those readers who were stumbling over heretical teachings.

John's advice coincides with the second most important commandment given in Matthew 22:39: "Love your neighbor as yourself." What does this mean for you? How can you love others and help them avoid stumbling?

TRUTH I WILL FOCUS ON TODAY

_____

_____

_____

_____

MY PRAYER

_____

_____

_____

_____

DAY 2

Scripture: 1 CORINTHIANS 6:19–20

Don't you realize that your body is the temple of the Holy Spirit, who lives in you and was given to you by God? You do not belong to yourself, for God bought you with a high price. So you must honor God with your body.

DEVOTIONAL THOUGHT

There are many reasons why we consider making changes in our lives: to live longer and healthier, to be a better parent for our kids, or a better spouse—to name a few. We do this because we love those people and don't want our years with them cut short. But Paul suggests another compelling reason: to honor God. Honoring God is a way of showing love for Him and to reflect appreciation for His sacrifice.

In the verse preceding this passage, Paul urged his readers to honor God by fleeing from sexual sin. But honoring God can also mean taking care of your body in general. How does "honor God with your body" play out in your life?

TRUTH I WILL FOCUS ON TODAY

_____

_____

_____

_____

MY PRAYER

_____

_____

_____

_____

DAY 3

Scripture: **1 TIMOTHY 4:15**

Give your complete attention to these matters. Throw yourself into your tasks so that everyone will see your progress.

DEVOTIONAL THOUGHT

What's the first quality of a leader that comes to your mind? Charismatic personality? Winning looks? Opinionated? The apostle Paul urged Timothy, a young leader, to value *diligence*. Throughout 1 Timothy 4 Paul advises Timothy to be diligent about warning believers about false teachers (verses 1–6), to avoid wasting time arguing over unimportant issues (verse 7), to preach and teach (verses 11–14), and to lead by example (verse 12).

This is a "clean your plate" approach to tasks, with love as the motivator. A loving, diligent, and committed leader inspires people far more than someone who merely delegates from a comfortable, superior position.

To which tasks do you give your wholehearted attention? What changes do you need to make to have the kind of diligence Paul describes?

TRUTH I WILL FOCUS ON TODAY

_____

_____

_____

_____

MY PRAYER

_____

_____

_____

_____

DAY 4

Scripture: TITUS 2:7

And you yourself must be an example to them by doing good works of every kind. Let everything you do reflect the integrity and seriousness of your teaching.

DEVOTIONAL THOUGHT

Paul mentored the leaders of the new churches that he helped start. Here he explains how Titus, a convert through Paul's ministry, can lead the young men in his own community.

Paul's description of leadership isn't exceptionally popular in our culture. Instead, we have a "say-it-for-the-sound bite" or "fake-it-for-the cameras" approach to leadership. We sometimes value looks and charisma over diligence and integrity. But Paul's description comes from the model of servant leadership and integrity in ministry that Jesus set for His disciples (see, for example, John 13 and Luke 4:16–21, 39–44). Is this your model of leadership? What leaders in your community model integrity? How can you encourage them as Paul encouraged Titus?

TRUTH I WILL FOCUS ON TODAY

_____

_____

_____

_____

MY PRAYER

_____

_____

_____

_____

DAY 5

Scripture: 1 TIMOTHY 4:12

Don't let anyone think less of you because you are young. Be an example to all believers in what you say, in the way you live, in your love, your faith, and your purity.

DEVOTIONAL THOUGHT

When Timothy's maturity as a leader was called into question, his spiritual father, the apostle Paul, was ready with advice, just as a good dad would be. His advice boils down to "lead by example." If Timothy exemplified purity, faith, and love, no one would question his maturity for long.

As a young leader, Jesus provided the ultimate example of love, faith, and purity. Jesus' wisdom often silenced His harshest critics. His life is the reason why Paul could urge Timothy to "be an example to all believers."

Think of the people who were role models for you. What characteristics made the deepest impression upon you? In what ways does your life reflect those characteristics?

TRUTH I WILL FOCUS ON TODAY

_____

_____

_____

_____

MY PRAYER

_____

_____

_____

_____

DAY 6

Scripture: 1 CORINTHIANS 10:33–11:1

I, too, try to please everyone in everything I do. I don't just do what is best for me; I do what is best for others so that many may be saved. And you should imitate me, just as I imitate Christ.

DEVOTIONAL THOUGHT

Paul is not urging the believers in Corinth to "look at me, look at me," as a young child would harp in a bid to gain a parent's attention. Nor is he advocating co-dependent people pleasing as a way of life. By imitating Jesus' way of life, Paul was showing that his focus was on Jesus, rather than on himself. This gave Paul the freedom to boldly love others. And loving others meant leading them to Jesus.

It is said that "imitation is the sincerest form of flattery," but Paul encourages behavior beyond flattery. He advocates a lifestyle that is compelling and contagious, rather than static or fear inducing. Is your imitation of Christ contagious?

TRUTH I WILL FOCUS ON TODAY

_____

_____

_____

_____

MY PRAYER

_____

_____

_____

_____

DAY 7

Scripture: 2 CORINTHIANS 12:19

Perhaps you think we're saying these things just to defend ourselves. No, we tell you this as Christ's servants, and with God as our witness. Everything we do, dear friends, is to strengthen you.

DEVOTIONAL THOUGHT

Ever feel you had to justify your words or actions? Perhaps you've felt that way after your teenager reacted negatively to a reproof or when a friend rebuked you for giving him or her a hard truth. Paul could relate. After sending letters of reproof to the Corinthian believers, Paul's only defense was to assure them of his love for them. "This is for your own good," he says in effect. We call this tough love, which isn't a valentine approach where everything is sugarcoated.

Loving others sometimes involves speaking the "truth in love" (Ephesians 4:15). This doesn't guarantee, however, that the recipient of the truth will listen with perfect acceptance and maturity. Has this been your experience? If not, how can you prepare now to show tough love to others?

TRUTH I WILL FOCUS ON TODAY

_____

_____

_____

_____

MY PRAYER

_____

_____

_____

_____

WEEKLY PROGRESS AND GOALS

- ❖ Current weight: _____
- ❖ Pounds lost this week: _____

NEW INSIGHTS

- ❖ About myself:

_____

_____

- ❖ From Scripture:

_____

_____

- ❖ About weight loss:

_____

_____

PLAN FOR NEXT WEEK

- ❖ Personal issue to focus on:

_____

_____

- ❖ Biblical truth to live out:

_____

_____

- ❖ Food to eliminate or restrict for the week:

_____

_____

- ❖ Exercise goals:

_____

_____

Notes

NOTES

NOTES

NOTES

NOTES

NOTES

NOTES

NOTES

NOTES

NOTES